Post-Traumatic Stress
– Not a Life Sentence

(Viewing Trauma and its Effects, through a Resilience Lens)

Nola Anne Hennessy

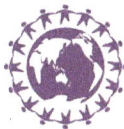

Serenidad® Consulting

This book may be ordered through booksellers, purchased directly from the publisher at www.serenidadconsulting.com/buy-our-books, and also by contacting the publisher directly at:

Serenidad Consulting Pty Ltd
PO Box 881
Sanctuary Cove QLD 4212
Australia

Email: enquiry@serenidadconsulting.com
www.serenidadconsulting.com/contact-us/

ISBN: 978-0-9943951-1-5 (sc)
ISBN: 978-0-9943951-2-2 (e)

Australian National Library CIP

The opinions expressed in this work are solely those of the author and are complemented by the author's professional and personal experiences. The author does not dispense medical advice or prescribe the use of any particular technique as a form of treatment for a condition, and advises that a qualified physician, rehabilitation provider and/or counsellor must be consulted by the reader where such circumstances warrant.

The intent of the author is only to offer information of a general nature to help the reader in the understanding of and recovery from trauma, and the development or enhancement of resilience. In the event the reader uses any of the information in this book for his/herself, which is the reader's constitutional and/or legal right, the author and the publisher assume no responsibility for the reader's decisions or actions, or the consequences of such.

Cover Design by: The Author

Serenidad Consulting Pty Ltd, 2/28/2017

CONTENTS

DEDICATION

This book is dedicated to my late Grandmother, Edna Daisy Jones. A woman who embodied and taught compassion, patience, warmth, forgiveness, love and understanding. I was blessed to have Edna Daisy Jones in my life from 1957 to 1989 and she will always be remembered by me as not only "Grandma", but also the best role model 'mom' a person could wish for.

Her loyalty to me never wavered, her kind love never waned, and her capacity to nurture and keep safe never faltered.

INTRODUCTION

Over the last few years many people and organizations have been keen to see me release this book, not the least because it provides a non-military-veteran perspective to living life after trauma. The fact that I am a happy and strong woman, is also another element that enables the subject of post-trauma recovery to be explored more fully and you will see throughout this book that I continually encourage people to think holistically about this important topic.

I bring to this book my knowledge and wisdom gained over more than 50 years since my first experience with a traumatic event; lengthy and discernment-based research; post-graduate qualifications in clinical hypnotherapy, human behaviours and various remedial therapies; and the resilience-building lessons I've learned and applied. I also bring direct experience working with, and knowing, military veterans who have been conditioned and programmed by their employers and/or the veteran health 'system' to believe that they will never recover from the impacts of the traumatic events they've survived.

However, this book is not about me, it's about you. Through my experiences surviving, recovering from and then learning to thrive after trauma, and closely observing and assisting/treating/supporting others who've been traumatized, I can write about this topic factually and without pride or prejudice.

My *sole intent* in writing this book is to help, empower and inspire trauma survivors. Whilst those on the periphery (counsellors, family members, medical and other health practitioners, rehabilitation providers etc.) will hopefully gain a better perspective of trauma and its effects, this book is not written for them. Unless they have experienced a traumatic event themselves, with all due courtesy to them, they will *never* understand what you are or have been going through.

I've lived through many different kinds of traumatic events since my early childhood and these are summarized in the last (optional-read) chapter titled "A Personal Reflection....". Whilst I've provided examples and context throughout the book, to help explain certain things based on my own experiences, the last chapter is optional because it's not necessary for you to understand *my* life history with trauma in order to improve outcomes for *you*.

By virtue of me living the life I have, I see this book as a way to share powerful information for the greater benefit of others. I wish you well in your journey of recovery and healing.

CHAPTER 1

Traumatic events and how they shape lives

In early 2013 one of my companies launched a couple of key seminars in Australia – one on "Building Community Resilience in Countering Violent Extremism", and the other one on "Post-Traumatic Stress – Not a Life Sentence". The latter was the first time that I am aware of where any person or entity had publicly advocated for post-traumatic stress symptoms to be seen as *fixable*.

By 2015 former President George W. Bush was quoted in The Washington Post[i], as stating (in reference to post-traumatic stress) "It's an injury....it's treatable". For military members and veterans it's also good that General Peter Chiarelli, US Army (Retired), has advocated the dropping of the 'D'[ii], as this appears to be the first major step for the USA military in de-stigmatizing and de-labelling post-traumatic stress.

However, as written in a blog article published in July 2015[iii], dropping the 'D' (i.e. the label of "disorder") is only a start. For too long post-traumatic stress symptoms have been labelled as a psychiatric condition which, based on my own research and experiences, I say they are not. For too long this topic has been whispered about but not openly addressed, and its sufferers pigeon-holed or conditioned to put-up-and-shut-up, perhaps for the sake of convenience. It's been one of those "too hard" topics that people appear loathe to talk about with positivity, tackle, and 'stay the course' to resolve.

Exposure to traumatic events and their aftermath impacts are not new phenomena. Traumatic events have been occurring at least as long as there have been humans around to experience them, and talk or write about them. Evidence is said to exist of humans recording their responses to traumatic events as early as 600 B.C., when traumas most often spoken about then involved the reactions of soldiers in combat. However by the 17th and 18th Centuries A.D. reporting on the impacts of traumatic events such as major fires, plagues and famine, had become common place. As authors, poets, sculptors and painters chose their art forms to illustrate and explain trauma, so too societies had begun to feel more comfortable to start talking about traumas suffered as a result of extreme events – extreme in the context that the events had exposed people to the very *extremes of normality*.

Yet, rightly or wrongly, in the 21st Century A.D. trauma and post-traumatic stress symptom discussions, coupled with the push by so many to perpetuate the case that post-trauma symptoms will never abate, have resulted in a key focus remaining on the military. It has been a long-held perception that only the military has more frequent exposure to situations which pose a threat to emotional and mental wellbeing. Perhaps this focus on the military is because of the sheer number of wars and violent engagements, perhaps because military veterans feel like they've been let down, perhaps because news media frequently focus on military stories and ravages of war. However, it's a real pity that we don't see any advocacy of significance coming from other front line professions, except perhaps from firefighters and police, though the reason for this absence of loud advocacy could be manyfold.

No doubt the consequences of fighting wars or being in other warlike situations can be catastrophic for some, but the impacts of trauma, regardless of the type of trauma, are felt across all sectors of society and through all demographic layers. Ensuring the emotional and mental wellbeing of any non-military front-line workers - emergency response personnel, police, health workers involved in direct patient care, and humanitarian workers involved in community rebuilding, for example - is no less important than for the military.

Likewise is the wellbeing of families and individuals living in, for example, traumatized communities or extreme situations. These people are just as important to protect and assist as the military and other professional front-line groups.

Only now are we beginning to acknowledge, and have at least some preliminary dialogue about, the impacts of traumatic events on police, emergency response personnel, refugees, communities in war zones, orphaned children, and victims of crime or domestic violence. Only now are we facing up to the fact that trauma = trauma = trauma, and traumatic events can occur everywhere in our world, in any context and at any time.

By the early 1990's traumatic events were starting to be recognized for the impacts they could create, however prior to that time there was little, if any, tangible action taken to intervene and provide critical incident first aid to the people affected at or by the event's 'scene'. Health practitioners long recognized that people's behaviour could alter after being involved in or witnessing a traumatic event, but psychiatric 'disorder' labels were still the only way to provide some context to the stressors introduced by, and symptoms arising in people after, a traumatic event.

By the late 1990's critical incident stress debriefings (CISDs) were both encouraged and welcomed, especially in communities and with workers exposed to traumatic events. In Australia for instance, CISDs had started being seen as a viable and useful option to provide immediate allied health support to communities and individuals after extreme events.

One particular Australian incident that pivoted the need for CISDs and immediate counselling-style support to trauma survivors, was the catastrophic landslide that occurred at Thredbo, in Australia's alpine and ski resort region. For many decades thousands had come every year, through all seasons, to enjoy Australia's highest mountain and its surrounding majestic landscapes. Thredbo and its satellite ski resorts were very popular

- similar places to what you would experience in any well-known ski-fields region around the world.

At that time the Snowy Mountains region in Australia had a very close knit mountain community where families knew families for generations and even strangers pitched-in and helped when help was needed. Even though spread across many thousands of kilometres the mountain folk in this bottom corner of New South Wales had one thing in common – an ability to survive severe cold weather in winter and raging bushfires in summer.

In July 1997, just before midnight and at the height of the skiing season in Australia's winter, the ski village was full with visitors and staff, and most people were asleep. Starting with a smaller breakaway section above one lodge, many thousands of tonnes of earth, together with buildings and part of the Alpine Way roadway, moved downhill at ever increasing speed. The massive slide took out a second lodge (housing most of the later deceased) and exposed not only an underground stream, which made search and rescue almost impossible, but also made all areas below the point of the original break in the landscape, highly vulnerable and unstable for at least the first 10 hours.

This natural disaster left only one survivor (Stuart Diver), whose 65+ hour long rescue from underneath snow, soil and rubble was watched and cheered on by millions on television. The landslide took 18 lives, including Stuart's wife whose body he laid next to for almost the whole time he was awaiting rescue. Aside from severe hypothermia Stuart sustained a range of life-threatening injuries and his other non-visible (emotional) injuries were only for *him* to truly know.

Stuart is regarded by many of his rescuers as having demonstrated remarkable mental endurance and determination - for the injuries he sustained, the support he gave to his wife while she was still alive, and the time he waited to be rescued. Stuart's inner strength was significant to his survival, as was the careful management of his physical and psychological condition, by the medical personnel supporting him during his rescue.

"Bob Garven, the Salvation Army captain seconded to the New South Wales Fire Brigades, says Diver's survival made a big difference to the healing of the scars of the rescue crews, and the nation.

"I remember going to bed at 1am the night before he was found," says Garven. "The temperature was below freezing and it looked like there was no chance of finding anyone alive. My pager went off at 6am to say they had found someone alive.

"It changed the whole atmosphere for everybody. Rescuers are motivated by saving lives, not body recovery. The personnel were becoming very depressed. But getting someone out alive meant they could finish the job knowing they had done their best and not lost everything.

"I think it affected the whole nation that way. People had been watching for days on television. Instead of talking about a terrible tragedy there was something positive and a sign of hope.""[iv]

The Thredbo Landslide remains the worst 'landslide' disaster in Australia's history and left scars on both the landscape and in the lives of many people. CISDs were undertaken on site for many days during the rescue and after the retrieval activities had ended. A range of other psychological support services were offered, by various members of the local and surrounding health services, for quite a long period.

Aside from Stuart's recovery and return to the mountain, some other good things that came out of this event were Australia's improvements to emergency management protocols and procedures, and the recognition that a coordinated and structured approach to emergency management was necessary. And it is this aspect, looking for the good that can come out of even the worst adversity, that is so vital to people being able to continue walking forward in life[v] after a traumatic event is over.

For many Australians, what made this catastrophic event difficult to fathom was the long-held belief that the mountain was as solid as a rock and that, perhaps because Australia is an 'old' landscape in geological terms, many believed nothing so devastating could possibly happen. The July 1997 event left pretty much the whole country in shock and, as the hours passed before rescue efforts could start, surprise turned to frustration and anger for many on the scene who were standing ready to help but were being told to hold back.

Stuart's rescue, and the recovery of the deceased, were hampered and delayed by a number of factors, not the least was the concern that further landslides would occur and potentially claim the lives of the dozens of first responders and support workers involved on site. For many rescue workers who were there, the mere act of having to 'wait' for the call to action may well have contributed to their own trauma at having to witness the events that unfolded. Yet, these rescuers didn't rate any particular public mention, regarding the impacts to them, so the general public remain none-the-wiser about the knock-on or collateral damage that can be done during and immediately after an event has passed.

In 1997 I lived only 120 kilometres from Thredbo in a small rural town. I was particularly keen to see post-trauma support provided to the communities affected because I had not only led the publicly funded community health services in the very region some years earlier, by that stage I was also consulting part-time (including on government community health management practices), and running a private clinic, counselling and providing remedial therapies support to clients, many of whom had been traumatized.

I also personally knew many people who, with specialist industrial skills (like concrete cutting) or paramedic training, were deployed to support search, rescue and retrieval efforts, and assist in the lengthy clean up after all the deceased were recovered from the rubble. Some of these workers refused to speak of what they saw, even with their own families, while some needed to talk about what they saw and did, or weren't allowed to do to help (due to the safety and stability concerns of the site), for many, many years afterwards.

****

Twenty years on from Stuart Diver's survival and the events that unfolded over many days and weeks in the Thredbo and surrounding communities, things are different. The now has been directly shaped by the event(s) of the past. Around the world, the realities of life in 2017 mean that potentially traumatic events now (unfortunately) include such things as man-made humanitarian crises, terrorist-related incidents, human trafficking and slavery, massacres (regardless of the weapon of choice), and even bullying.

What we expect to see or hear about regularly now has, unfortunately, gone way beyond what we have previously known to be typical traumatic events: things such as major crimes, death or serious injury or long term incapacity, rape and incest, abuse (of any kind), any life-threatening situation, an unplanned and extreme impact event which occurs with little warning (e.g. industrial, rail, plane, vessel/ship or motor vehicle accidents), war and warlike situations, violent incidents resulting in murder and serious injury, financial collapse, abandonment or wilful neglect (particularly of children), a drug overdose, and environmental disasters.

The impact of a traumatic event can be measured in any number of ways - human, financial, reputational, physical/environmental, civil, security, and societal governance terms; and the outcomes of a traumatic event can be catastrophic, at so many levels, with the recovery being long, or seemingly impossible to achieve.

When it comes to the human cost of traumatic events, what I find most concerning is that there is currently no evidence (that I'm aware of) to demonstrate that those who now *claim to be experts* in how to "treat" and "manage" symptomatology associated with the actual trauma, have ever personally experienced an event sufficiently excessive to cause a post-trauma response in themselves. The 'experts' are, in reality, merely observers of the experts, for the true experts are the ones who've survived the traumatic event.

The second part of my concern is that whilst ever the health practitioner (or the actual trauma recipient[1]) is "treating" and "managing" just the symptoms, and not addressing and removing root causes, they are blocking the best path to full and complete rehabilitation and recovery of the trauma rehabilitee (i.e. the one undergoing the rehabilitation post-trauma). When a trauma rehabilitee acknowledges root causes for their injury/ies they are automatically empowered with information sufficient to

---

[1] who from the point of trauma through to full healing is no different, in recovery terms, to any other injury/illness rehabilitee

enable them to heal. Under the "treat and manage" scenario the cycle of symptoms will undoubtedly continue, which leaves the trauma rehabilitee in a dependent, 'losing' state of mind.

This situation becomes further exacerbated when the trauma rehabilitee receives an ongoing "disability" pension or payment – the check (cheque) that arrives regularly in the mail that reminds them each time "we think you're disabled". Some form of rehabilitation support payment may be warranted for a period, however I truly believe making a trauma rehabilitee forever dependent on a disability' compensation system does nothing to strengthen their self-esteem or provide proactive tools for their empowerment to affect positive change in their lives. The whole reason for rehabilitating someone is to restore them to whatever level of normality that the rehabilitee truly wants to achieve, and restore them holistically – physically, mentally, emotionally and spiritually. A good rehabilitation program will assist a rehabilitee to restore themselves at a spiritual level and also improve their self-esteem.

Some of you might say it's OK for your medical advisor or health practitioner not to have any personal experience with trauma and therefore be coming from a position of only theory because, as we all know, to become a specialist in certain fields (e.g. brain surgery) you actually don't have to undergo it yourself to know how to be a good surgeon. I would agree that in some professions there are a few good practitioners with a wealth of patient-based experiential learning (i.e. knowledge arising from their patients' conditions) who are successful in either curing or assisting their patients to a level of recovery. I have no doubt this happens every day. However I do believe these practitioners are the exception to the rule.

For the trauma rehabilitees who are tossed aside in the "we can't help you anymore" pile, we simply don't hear enough about them to know just how many could well have been shown a different path to healing and recovery, rather than remain a statistic at the negative end of the spectrum (the "almost fixed" patients, the "90%ers").

Another part of my concern is in relation to responses to trauma. The potential for someone to exhibit post-trauma emotional responses for short or long periods, and the uniqueness of their symptomatology, is completely equal to the uniqueness of that individual. No two humans will respond to a traumatic event and the stressors involved, or perhaps go on to exhibit post-trauma or even post-traumatic stress symptoms, in exactly the same way. One person's response to trauma might *appear* to be the same type of response as someone else is exhibiting, but to say that one person's response, or the symptoms of post-traumatic stress appearing in that person, are *identical* across all humans is as false as saying that an injury from which the person *appears not to heal*, automatically creates a disorder or disability in that person.

By its very nature post-trauma symptomatology is always going to be a moving phenomenon. Symptoms are, after all, subjective and based on the perception of the *individual* (see Chapter 2 for some relevant definitions). In fact the reliance to date on labelling something a disorder simply accentuates the notion that a disorder is permanent and not fixable. A dis-order can be finite in its duration, no differently than dis-ease can, and usually is, finite in its duration. By comparison to centuries past, there are very few dis-eases that modern medicine can't treat and/or cure. And, suffice to say, there would be even more cures available if those in positions of power (whose personal wealth may well rely on them staying silent about known cures), chose to walk the integrity path and reveal the cure secrets that they hold so close.

In any field of human physiology and health management there are the experts who have the theoretical knowledge but no first-hand experience in the subject matter, and then there are those who have the theoretical knowledge coupled with direct and relevant experience. I advocate that the latter are better placed to inform rehabilitees about effective treatment and healing regimes. I have respect for medical professionals who treat and guide their 'patients' holistically but, again, these highly alert and think-outside-the-box practitioners are few and far between in our modern world of medicine. Most medical practitioners will happily stay within the theoretical model they were taught in university, not the least because their medical malpractice insurance would probably not support a claim if it was found that they deviated from standard clinical practices or advocated for more holistic treatment regimes.

Any decent rehabilitation program should always, repeat always, have an end goal of restoring the person to as normal a state of health as possible. There is no *valid* reason for the medical profession to see post-traumatic stress symptoms as anything more than a transitory state for the person affected. Furthermore, post-trauma responses don't always progress into a more prolonged and severe post-traumatic stress set of symptoms. The individual's personal experience with the traumatic event, coupled with any resilience already developed in the past, will determine *how* they respond to the event and manage their emotions and thoughts, and for *how short or long a period.*

To immediately pigeon-hole, box or label a person as having a disorder *just because* they exhibit symptoms seen on the medical profession's checklist for post-traumatic stress, is naïve at best and arrogant at worst. Are mental health and physical health diagnostic manuals so perfect that they lack errors, inconsistencies and omissions? During my research for this book, and previously in other contexts, I have found so many contradictions and ambiguities it adds even more value to what this book is about. By saying that a set of symptoms listed in a diagnostic manual is the only viable set of symptoms with which to judge someone's state of health belies the whole notion of the evolving sciences. Just because a symptom is currently listed in a diagnostic manual doesn't mean that it will always be there or that other symptoms aren't valid. At some point in time a symptom in that list may be removed, when it's found to lack relevance. At another time another symptom might be added. It's always going to be a moving feast.

Symptoms rely on information from the individual, and his/her perceptions and experiences. Therefore, in reality, a medical text, dictionary or case study is only relevant *for a period in time*, and will only ever be in the context of the actual 'patients' who shared their symptoms, for the improved knowledge of the medical profession.

In my first book, *No Boxing Allowed,* which was written in 2005-7 and first published in 2009, I am passionate in advocating that change in the medical profession needs to occur. The general populous of medical practitioners are doing nothing short of *practicing* on their patients and, to add insult to injury, rarely do they really learn and apply any lessons. The medical script-book (no pun intended) is how they run their "practice" and likely why some forget the oath of 'first do no harm', willy-nilly making life altering decisions and imposing their opinion on their patients. The patient becomes their experiment and, in reality, medical advances or changes are only achieved when a breakthrough piece of information is validated by enough evidence and *allowed* to be released into broader practice. Testing and experimentation, including on people, is key to that success.

In this book I advocate that moving away from mental health treatment and dependency cycles, and viewing lenses, are critical to enabling and empowering people after trauma. Focusing more on human physiology and how the body naturally adapts to normal stressors, including the General Adaptation Syndrome (GAS) that is a fundamental component of the system required for human survival and recovery, is going to deliver better long-term outcomes and a greater understanding of the body's innate ability to heal itself. In my own experience, I know the Self Intelligence [vi] -based model is a far more powerful approach to aid recovery and healing, and development of resilience in individuals post-trauma.

In researching for and writing this book I have reflected long and hard on my own experiences. I know without doubt that the human impact of traumatic events deserve our focus, not in mental health treatment terms but in *injury prevention* terms. I further believe that complete healing from post-traumatic stress symptoms can be achieved, through choosing a path of recovery, repair, resilience and empowerment.

A change in thinking to the positive and visualizing a 'best-case' result, automatically empowers those who've endured trauma to take control of their health and wellbeing outcomes and focus on achieving a fully healed state, where this is physiologically possible.

CHAPTER 2

Back to Basics – factual terms and definitions, and how to make sense of it all

This chapter is designed to not only simplify the way you look at trauma and its impacts, but also to set the baseline for the terms used throughout this book. Establishing a baseline is always helpful when you have to compare things, and by having some clear definitions this allows consistency to prevail and helps remove the likelihood of ambiguity or confusion. All terms and definitions have been sourced from publicly available information or from my private library of reference material. Explanation or clarification is provided where I believe it's necessary, however my main goal is to simplify.

During my comparative research activities for this book I found a significant range of inconsistent, contradictory and ambiguous information publicly available through the world-wide web. It is for this reason that I have weeded out the information that I think could confuse you, in order to present the current facts in as easy-to-understand language as possible.

Other than for pure definitions obtained from the Merriam-Webster Dictionary, noted in the table as (MW), the Oxford Dictionary, noted as (O), or the Cambridge Dictionary, noted as (C), each specific reference from a public or published source is appropriately referenced as an end note to enable you to further research and understand these terms in the context of your own life experiences with trauma. All quotations taken from website-based sources are true and correct as at February 2017, therefore any amendments made at source by the owners of the website pages, subsequent to this book's production, must not be taken to replace the words described here. As I mentioned earlier, this book sets a baseline from which to move forward. I draw a line in the sand so that everyone can start from the same point of understanding - I believe this is the most logical way to approach the topic of trauma, and the mental health management model that so many practitioners still want to push.

My personal and professional library consists of reference books, government-supplied regulatory information, practitioner manuals, educator/trainer reference material, student workbooks and best practice methodologies, most of which I've developed and used over more than three decades. Since my first appointment to lead Federal Government clients in the field of ICT and ergonomics in 1984, I've conducted a successful private remedial therapies and counselling clinic during the 1990's and, from the early 1990's, managed, advised and consulted on, facilitated and also educated about community health, best practice health and safety, sound risk management, and sustainable return-to-work of injured clients. Through all of these decades the one thing that remained the center of my focus was improving outcomes for the 'individual'. Community health services, health and safety management, injury management and rehabilitation is all about people, after all.

Some of you may recognize the acronym KISS. In this book when I say KISS it means 'Keep It Simple and Strategic'. This is a phrase I've taught many times during my organization's Great Leadership™ training and coaching sessions and I can guarantee the reception of my version of KISS is far more positive. Not the least because it focuses people on strategy (which generally points you forward in your thinking rather than backward, and produces a structured way of doing things) and also, because keeping things simple is critical to understanding and navigating the nuances of trauma and injury management.

My recommendation to you is to remain aware that information that originates in the world of medicine is changing all the time, and mental health is not a recognized field of science. *Science* is about gathering information through observation, to formulate theories, to then create knowledge. *Pure science* is concerned with simply gathering information for the purpose of knowledge rather than applying that knowledge in practical terms, whereas *applied science* is the practical application of scientific theory and laws.

When it comes to the sciences, even the categories of science have changed over the years: from the earth, physical and life sciences to (now) what's referred to as the natural, social and formal sciences. Yet, despite these changes, three key things remain consistent:

- the scientific method: is a systematic and ordered approach to the gathering of data and the solving of a problem; most often expressed and tested in hypothesis terms. The hypothesis states the 'problem' as a factual starting point using (usually) minimal information available. From this point scientific experimentation is used to prove or disprove the hypothesis, drawn from observable results and, if proven correct, a scientific rationale (or evidence-based reason) can then be given for a proposed course of action. All in all, a very strategic approach as it is facts, not assumptions, that are used as the foundation for experimentation;

- scientific reasoning: is either deductive ('premise' or 'known principle'-based) or inductive (discovery and observation-based). *Deductive reasoning*, often referred to as top-down reasoning, leads from something known (predetermined) and general, to something specific and usually unknown (a prediction) and is most often applied to the scientific method noted above. *Inductive reasoning* involves the analysis of data (both qualitative and quantitative) and observation and examination of the practical 'problems' in their own context, rather than using a predetermined, theoretical basis. It is more a bottom-up reasoning, where assumptions not facts are tested;

- psychology and psychiatry are not science: in both the original and new 'science' categories, the absence of both of these disciplines of medicine, from the pure and applied sciences, is strikingly obvious.

It is relatively easy to apply the scientific method to the physical sciences such as physics and chemistry. However, in the life sciences (such as biology, zoology, physiology and botany) and earth sciences (such as geology and astronomy) because of the unique nature of the subject matter, the scientific method becomes not only less relevant, but also more difficult to achieve repetitive experimentation (and therefore proving or disproving something is unachievable).

In the context of helping people with their emotional responses post-trauma, what I have to question is how medical practitioners can apply such vigorous support to the fields of psychology and psychiatry, when there is no scientific proof that a mental health treatment regime does anything to fix (i.e. heal) a traumatized individual?

Furthermore, social science is often times misrepresented in order to encapsulate the behavioural sciences, however there is no formally recognized and factual basis for calling psychology, psychiatry and human behaviours, a science. Whilst a university can create a 'school' for such, and award a "science" degree after successful completion of the field of study, where is the proof that these tertiary studies are actually worthy of recognition as study in a field of *science*?

A degree in psychology or psychiatry may be worthy of professional recognition as say, a minimum qualification required for working as a clinician but, apart from that, who's to say the graduate is worthy of recognition as a science practitioner? When the professions themselves are still fighting for recognition and claiming a scientific basis for these academic fields of endeavour, to call psychiatry or psychology a science is like saying that a Chartered Accountant (CA) is a specialist of the accountancy sciences. In my opinion, both notions are as contradictory as each other and, I'm sure, have simply arisen as a result of there being no universally-recognized and empowered global entity for the advancement of the sciences; an entity that sets the international framework and standards for science, and is the foremost authority. Even the International Standards Organization [vii] (ISO) has not published a science standard that refers to any of the work practices of psychiatry and psychology (or accountancy for that matter).

The Diagnostic and Statistical Manual of Mental Disorders (DSM) now in its Fifth Edition (DSM-5) 2013, is the most commonly used and recognized (by psychiatrists, and other medical and mental health practitioners) reference manual for the diagnosis of a mental health condition. "Beginning 2000 work groups were formed to create a research agenda for the fifth major revision of *DSM* (*DSM–5*). These work groups generated hundreds of white papers, monographs, and journal articles, providing the field with a summary of the state of the science relevant to psychiatric diagnosis and letting it know where gaps existed in the current research, with hopes that more emphasis would be placed on research within those areas."[viii] I find it interesting the use of the words "a summary of the state of the science relevant to psychiatric diagnosis" as there is, on the referenced website, no mention of the field of 'science' that psychiatry is claimed to be based on. There is much talk of incorporating science into psychiatry, which I think is a good thing, but not of psychiatry being a science in its own right.

The DSM is informed by the World Health Organization's International Classification of Diseases (ICD), and in fact the ICD underwent significant changes as a direct result of World War II and input from the American Army [ix]. The ICD-10 includes information which "sets out internationally-agreed diagnostic criteria specifically designed for use when conducting research on mental and behavioural disorders. Deliberately restrictive, the criteria are intended to facilitate the selection of groups of individuals whose symptoms and other characteristics resemble each other in clearly stated ways, and thus to maximize the homogeneity of study groups and the comparability of findings in multicentre and international studies............................(the) disorders are described with the aim of stimulating the research needed to clarify their diagnostic relevance and allow their more precise classification."[x] Once again, an emphasis is placed on *research* and gaining a greater understanding (of mental health), not on the implementation of practical solutions or proven treatment regimes.

If I were to continue to research the number and content of court proceedings where so-called expert witness testimony has been refuted for having no factual basis in science, I could well earn myself a PhD in the subject. The mental health practitioners have been working hard for years to link scientific evidence to real-life practices, perhaps to help create a level of efficacy of and worthiness in their professional activities. When the testimony of such practitioners in a court room situation, can work to determine a person's life outcomes and influence an otherwise undecided jury, I would sincerely recommend the justices appointed to ensure accurate jury deliberations and decide rulings, pay more mind to what can be scientifically proven, rather than surmised.

So that you can appreciate the volume of information floating around the public domain, my background research for this book involved activities best summarized by these analogies: me fossicking to find a fine needle in a wet haystack; sifting through flour to find a single grain of powdered sugar; or (worse case) squeezing the BS out of the flood of useless information that lies on the WWW, to achieve at least a clean dry slate to work from. There is not only too much information out there, a lot of it is simply inaccurate, unverified and unreferenced.

From the point of view of accurate reference texts, I also recommend you remain aware that with every new 'discovery' the medical profession throws out many of its old medical precedents, and starts with the new. I mentioned this a little earlier when I was discussing the list of symptoms that doctors refer to. This practice of refreshment, whilst a good thing in that information is kept as current as possible, unfortunately feeds the ambiguities and contradictions that already exist between information sources, and will undoubtedly exacerbate the efficacy of data and information going forward.

Another rather important reason I chose to include this chapter is to share with you not only the meaning of key terms but also introduce the nuances associated. You may see immediate and clear contradictions in what you have been told, when compared to the definitions articulated below. And if those alarm bells create more dialogue with the people involved in your rehabilitation or support, then that's a good thing.

Further, I felt it important to de-stigmatize injuries to one's emotions, and particularly post-traumatic stress symptoms, so that those on the periphery who have previously chosen to criticize or belittle your response(s) to trauma, can now be handed an opportunity to educate-away their ignorance, and begin their own journey towards being fully compassionate and genuinely understanding.

The obvious, yet rarely discussed, divide in understanding between those who have endured and survived traumatic events, and those who have not, is cause enough. Ignorance breeds contempt, especially when the ignorant choose to keep their heads in the sand or not listen.

My long-held and unwavering belief is that people who've been delivered a traumatic event to endure, and physically survive if circumstances allow, are actually the stronger ones emotionally and mentally. A human being's journey in life is full of events, some in our control, some not. To get to the end of life and know that you've survived and thrived through the adversity created by a traumatic event can, when you see the positive side, be seen as a gift. Stuart Diver is a perfect example of a positive attitude being instrumental in not only surviving the actual event, but living a full and complete life afterwards.

I do believe you were chosen to endure and learn, by circumstances within and outside of your control, because the universe knew you were strong enough to handle the traumatic event(s) you have been through. I do believe that strong people are sent tests, to not only show them what they're capable of surviving, but also to enable them to be a positive example to others.

Why did Stuart Diver survive? Was it so that when he remarried he could become the rock for his new wife, who was diagnosed with cancer only weeks after their marriage? Or was it so that he could, against all the odds, have a beautiful daughter with his second wife and then, after yet another loss, raise his daughter in an environment where they both felt at home? Or was it both?

Ultimately, how you choose to progress your life after a traumatic event is always *your choice and in your control.*

Now to some important terms and definitions:

Term (noun)	Simple Definition and Accompanying Notes
disease	L, *dis* + Fr, *aise*, ease – 1. a condition of abnormal vital function involving any structure, part or system of an organism 2. a specific illness or disorder characterized by a recognizable set of signs or symptoms, attributable to heredity, infection, diet or environment.[xi]
disorder	L, *dis*, apart + *ordo*, rank - a disruption of or interference with normal functions or established systems e.g. mental disorder, nutritional disorder[xii] See also: interference; interferent; disruption, homeostasis
disruption (C)	an interruption in the usual way that a system, process or event works.
emotion	the affective (feeling) aspect of consciousness as compared with volition or cognition. Physiologic (human body) changes often occur with a marked change of emotions.[xiii] MW refers to: * affective as - relating to, arising from, or influencing feelings or emotions; and * emotion as - a state of feeling.

Term (noun)	Simple Definition and Accompanying Notes
event	In the context of risk management: the occurrence or change of a particular set of circumstances.[xiv] Other generic definitions: * (C) anything that happens, especially something important or unusual * (MW) something that happens (i.e. an occurrence) See also: traumatic, risk management, trauma
fight-or-flight response	when you are (or feel) threatened physically or emotionally, your sympathetic nervous system (SNS) brings about the "flight-or-fight" response to help you cope with the stressful situation. As organ stimulation occurs, key stress responses include from the: 1) Hypothalamus - part of the body's nervous system (which is built for speed) but also recognized as an endocrine organ because it produces several hormones which stimulate other endocrine organs. It has a two-fold function in the stress response. In the *alarm phase*, which is short-term, nerve impulses from the hypothalamus stimulate SNS target organs (including the Adrenal Medulla described below), to produce stress responses such as:

Term (noun)	Simple Definition and Accompanying Notes
	• increasing the heart rate and blood pressure; • causing the liver to convert glycogen to glucose and release glucose to the blood; • dilating the bronchioles; • decreasing digestive system activity; • decreasing urine output; • increasing alertness; and • changing blood flow patterns. In the *resistance phase* of the stress response, which is more prolonged, the hypothalamus secretes a hormone which stimulates the pituitary gland, which in turn stimulates other endocrine organs to release hormones to respond to the stressor in a range of ways including: • retention of sodium and water by the kidneys; • increasing blood volume and pressure; • hyperglycaemia; • causing proteins and fats to be broken down for energy; and • depressing inflammatory responses.[xv] 2) Adrenal Medulla – which literally pumps its two very similar hormones (adrenaline and noradrenaline – collectively referred to as catecholamines) into the bloodstream to enhance and prolong the effects of the neurotransmitters of the SNS. The effect of the catecholamines is to increase heart rate, blood pressure, and blood glucose levels, and dilate the lungs' small passageways. This results in more

Term (noun)	Simple Definition and Accompanying Notes
	oxygen and glucose in the blood, and faster circulation of the blood to the body's organs (important ones being the brain, heart and muscles). The body is thus better able to deal with a short-term stressor, whether the job at hand is to fight (given the inflammatory process) or make you more alert so you can think more clearly.
	The catecholamines prepare the body to cope with a brief, short-term stressful situation and cause the so-called *alarm stage* of the stress response.[xvi]
	3) Adrenal Cortex – which produces three major groups of steroid hormones (collectively called corticosteroids) two of which are fundamental players in the stress response:
	• mineralocorticoids, for regulating the mineral (or salt) content of the blood and helping manage blood volume and pressure; and
	• glucocorticoids, for promoting normal cell metabolism and helping the body resist *long-term stressors*, primarily by increasing blood glucose levels, assisting the breakdown of proteins and fats for energy; and helping depress the inflammatory response.[xvii]
	See also: stressor, GAS, homeostasis

Term (noun)	Simple Definition and Accompanying Notes
general adaptation syndrome (GAS)	the defence response of the body or the psyche, to injury or prolonged stress (exposure to stressors), consisting of an initial stage of shock or alarm reaction, followed by a stage of increasing resistance or adaptation, using the various defence mechanisms of the body or mind.[xviii] See also: stressor, fight-or-flight response, homeostasis
homeostasis	* a relative constancy in the internal environment of the body, naturally maintained by adaptive responses that promote healthy survival. Various sensing, feedback, and control mechanisms function to effect this steady state. Some of the functions controlled by homeostatic mechanisms are the heartbeat, haematopoiesis, blood pressure, body temperature, electrolyte balance, respiration and glandular secretion.[xix] * a state of body equilibrium; describes the body's ability to maintain a relatively stable internal environment even though the outside world is continually changing. Although the literal meaning is "unchanging" (*homeo* = the same; *stasis* = standing still), the term means that rather than the body being in an unchanged state, it is in a *dynamic* state of equilibrium, or a balance in which internal conditions change and vary, but always within relatively narrow limits. When you think of the fact that the body contains trillions of cells in nearly constant activity, and that remarkably little usually

Term (noun)	Simple Definition and Accompanying Notes
	goes wrong with it, one can appreciate the marvellous machine that the body is. Homeostasis is so important that most disease is regarded as a result of its disturbance, a condition called homeostatic imbalance. Such imbalances can affect a range of body systems including the respiratory, lymphatic, circulatory and endocrine.[xx] To help you visualize this, imagine a wavy horizontal line which peaks and troughs (like a sound wave would look) but constantly works to bring the line back into balance (horizontal) despite changes occurring outside of the line's control. Homeostasis is the balanced flat line and the body's response(s) to stressors produce the peaks and troughs. Note regarding therapeutic massage – these massage methods are simple and effective in producing responses mediated through the nervous system, the interaction with the endocrine system, the connective tissue, and the circulatory system. With an understanding of the physiologic effects of massage, it is hoped that individuals, in consultation with medical personnel, will consider the use of these very old and effective methods provided by trained massage professionals, in the development of conservative treatment plans for chronic pain and stress-induced disease processes, before resorting to more invasive measures. Therapeutic massage could play an important role in prevention programs by providing a natural mechanism to stimulate

Term (noun)	Simple Definition and Accompanying Notes
	the body to adjust to the stress of daily life and restore the natural homeostatic balance.[xxi] See also: GAS, stressor, resilience, disease, disorder
hormones	from a Greek word meaning "to arouse", they are the secretions of the endocrine glands, with the glands playing an essential role in maintaining homeostasis. As chemical substances secreted by cells, hormones are responsible for regulatory effects on certain (target) body parts or organs, including regulating the metabolic activity of other cells in the body. They arouse, or bring about their effects, primarily by altering cellular activity.[xxii]
illness	an unhealthy condition; an abnormal process in which aspects of the condition and function of a person are diminished or impaired compared with that person's previous condition.[xxiii]
illness experience	the five stage process of being ill: Phase 1 – experiencing a symptom; Phase 2 – assuming a sick role; Phase 3 – making contact for health care; Phase 4 – being dependent (a patient); and Phase 5 – recovering or being rehabilitated[xxiv]

Term (noun)	Simple Definition and Accompanying Notes
interference (MW)	a noun for the act or process of interfering or obstructing; something which interferes e.g. an obstruction. In other dictionaries, referred to as something that hinders, involves, impinges, encroaches, or opposes.
interferent	any chemical or physical phenomena that can interfere or disrupt a reaction or process.[xxv]
injury (MW)	hurt, damage or loss sustained.
psychosomatic	Gk, *psyche,* mind + *soma,* body 1. relating to, characterized by, or resulting from the interaction of the mind and the body 2. the expression of an emotional conflict through physical symptoms.[xxvi] Emotional distress exhibits as a physical symptom *for which the physical symptom has no known cause.* Examples of such physical symptoms (without the presence of a known physical cause) can include chest/back/abdominal pain, headache, nausea, stomach upset, oedema, numbness, cough, and constipation.
resilience	In medicine, nursing and allied health fields: L, *resilere,* to spring back the ability of a body to return to its original form after being stretched or

27

Term (noun)	Simple Definition and Accompanying Notes
	compressed.[xxvii] In the context of emotional resilience: * (MW) an ability to recover from and adjust easily to misfortune or change. Other generic definitions: * (O) the capacity to recover quickly from difficulties; toughness. * (MW) the ability to become strong, healthy and successful again after something bad happens. * (C) able to quickly return to a previous good condition. See also: homeostasis, GAS, fight-or-flight response, stressor
risk management	coordinated activities to direct and control the individual with regard to risk. Involves the systematic process of: • establishing the context of the risk; • performing a risk assessment (risk identification, risk analysis and risk evaluation); and • treating the risk. *Risk* is often characterized by reference to potential **events** and **consequences**, or a combination of these. Likewise risk is often expressed in terms of a combination of the consequences of an event (including changes in circumstances) and the

Term (noun)	Simple Definition and Accompanying Notes
	associated **likelihood** of occurrence.[xxviii] Important Note – As with all international standards, ISO 31000:2009 can be used by any public, private or community enterprise, association, group or individual. All the different kinds of users of ISO 31000:2009 are referred to by the general term "organization". For ease of comprehension the word organization is replaced by "individual".
stressor	* anything that causes wear and tear on the body's physical or mental resources.[xxix] * any stimulus that directly or indirectly causes the hypothalamus to initiate stress-reducing responses, such as the fight or flight response.[xxx] Important note - the individual's response(s) to stressor(s) are managed via the GAS and therefore directly contingent on the overall healthy condition of the individual. See also: GAS, fight-or-flight response, homeostasis, illness
symptom	Gk, *symptoma*, that which happens a subjective indication of a disease or a change in condition as perceived by the patient. Primary symptoms are <u>intrinsically associated with</u> the disease process. Secondary symptoms are a <u>consequence</u> of the disease process.[xxxi]

Term (noun)	Simple Definition and Accompanying Notes
symptomatology	the science of symptoms of disease in general, or of the symptoms of a specific disease.[xxxii]
trauma	in its singular form, trauma is the Greek (Gk) word for "wound". Can be used as a combining word, e.g. neurotrauma, and used to describe one or both of the following: 1. a physical injury caused by violent or disruptive action[xxxiii] 2. psychic injury resulting from severe emotional shock.[xxxiv]
traumatic	pertaining to an injury, usually a serious or unexpected injury.[xxxv]

You've probably noticed I didn't include the DSM's definitions of post-traumatic stress here. There's one reason for that – I want you to forget about viewing psychic trauma through a mental health lens. The DSM looks at post-traumatic stress as an anxiety-related issue and I know, and you know, "anxiety" **may or may not** be one of your post-trauma responses. Psychic trauma is about emotional injury, not mental injury. And an emotional injury can result from or follow a physical injury, both of which have a root cause in the traumatic event.

It entirely depends on the individual how the after effects of a traumatic event will manifest in them at a physiological level. The individual's upbringing, adaptability, current level of emotional resilience, mindset, general health and fitness, self-awareness, plus (and perhaps most importantly) *what's going on in the individual's life at the time of the event*, all play a part in determining how the trauma will be navigated, and how quickly recovery can be achieved and normality resumed.

You may also wonder why I've included so much information about the body's stress response. The reason for this is that everything in the body is interlinked/interdependent. Understanding the interdependencies of and cause-and-effect relationship between organs and how they function will help you to gain a more holistic view of yourself. Some may advocate that certain organs are surplus to requisite (e.g. the appendix). Well, that may be the case from a doctor's perspective, however I'm of the opinion that each component of the human body is placed there for a reason and to understand how the body works is far better than remaining ignorant. When we know our bodies, so too can we begin to listen to our bodies.

Further, it's important to start (if you haven't already) understanding the very significant link between emotions, the mind and the body. In my first two books (*No Boxing Allowed* and *From Pre-Menstrual Syndrome to Positive Mental Attitude)*, I talk about the mind-body connection and how your body will manifest what your mind believes. This correlates to the notion of 'your life will manifest as you believe it will', simply because the mind is *such* a powerful tool and ally which can aid your recovery and healing from injury and illness, whether trauma-related or not.

'Mind-over-matter' is also an often-used term in the context of the getting over an event or an injury, however because it is often used to brush away someone's symptoms and at times without any regard for the severity of the person's responses, exploring it to any further degree here is, in my opinion, not going to add any significantly greater value to the topic of trauma and its effects, and developing resilience.

CHAPTER 3

Understanding the impact of a trauma in experience terms, not mental health terms

A traumatic event is typically unexpected, uncontrolled, and extreme. At an emotional level, these kinds of events generally shock, threaten and/or overwhelm an individual's sense of safety and security. They may, and generally do, leave the individual feeling vulnerable, helpless and/or insecure in their environment. And, in many instances the individual may experience or witness an event that is life-threatening to them or another, or actually involves the death of one or more people.

Abrupt and short-term traumatic events, lasting a few minutes to a number of days, can include natural events and those involving human choice (intentional or accidental). Natural disasters include events such as tornados, earthquakes, avalanches, hurricanes, cyclones, floods and sinkholes. Human-made (and usually) unplanned incidents include such things as vehicle and plane crashes, building fires, explosions, workplace injuries or deaths, collateral damage to private citizens and communities during warfighting, personal health events such as a heart attack or stroke, and so on. Human-made deliberate (intentional) acts

33

include such events as rape, gun violence, assault, terrorist bombings, robbery, abduction (kidnap), abandonment, and combat in a more general sense.

Sustained, repeated and longer-term traumatic events can result from the above abrupt events, however they are usually of a chronic, repetitive nature and involve ongoing exposure of the individual to the threat. These kinds of traumatic events are usually either natural or technological disasters, or human-made deliberate events and, like abrupt traumatic events, are non-uniform (heterogeneous) in nature. Natural and technological disasters usually include things like a nuclear reactor accidents, toxic spills, and environmental pollution, or can arise from poor workplace safety practices. Events arising from intentional human design include such things as being taken as a prisoner-of-war, domestic violence, child abuse (sexual or otherwise), refugee displacement or internment, human trafficking, invasion of a community or country, and so on.

How an individual responds to a traumatic event is entirely subjective and unique. No two individuals will respond in exactly the same way, even to the same event, because of all of the variable factors that go into the makeup of the individual (see more on this in Chapter 2). Hence why this book focuses on the 'individual', rather than seeing post-trauma symptoms and post-traumatic stress as something more generic.

Ultimately though, it's the word *trauma* that is most significant in understanding what happened to you and how to manage your response(s).

As defined in Chapter 2, *trauma* is the Greek word for injury. In medicine, trauma is seen as either a physical injury caused by violent or disruptive action, or a psychic injury resulting from severe emotional shock. Your management of and recovery post-trauma will be driven entirely by *how and to what degree the traumatic event has impacted you* – physical injury/ies, psychic injury, **or both**, and the severity of the injury/ies.

The approach to managing the *longer term* impacts of trauma, whether physical, psychic or both, is going to be different in many respects however, in managing the *immediate* impacts of the trauma the focus needs to remain on the commonality of trauma – i.e. whether the impacts are short or long term, you are still managing any injury.

You may be aware of the acronym that is used to help first aid students remember what to do in a stressful situation, where an event has occurred which results in injury to someone:– they follow the D.R.A.B.C. methodology as the first step in delivering first aid:

D – Danger

R – Response

A – Airway

B – Breathing

C – Circulation

Leaving aside the management of a physical injury, which is not the subject of this book even though it may be relative to a psychic injury, how the first aider (and this could be yourself if you're alone) manages the situation is helped along by asking some simple questions, as swiftly as possible. Targeted questions can help inform how the injured person may be responding to the situation at an emotional level and, in that context, we'll look at just the first two parts of D.R.A.B.C., the D and the R.

By using a yes/no process of elimination, the best and most likely the safest path for first aid management of the injured's emotional response to the event can then be chosen:

Danger – is danger still present? If so, what is causing the danger? Can the threat be removed or minimized? Can the person be moved somewhere safer? Can the person be supported emotionally whilst the danger is still present?

Response – is the injured person conscious and responsive to questions? Is the person exhibiting signs of emotional shock? Is the person lucid and alert? Is the person able to articulate how they feel?

Regardless of whether you are administering your own first aid, or someone else is, the aim of the first aider is always to stay calm, caring, and compassionate, and make confident decisions. If you're being attended to by a first aider, or being a first aider to someone else less traumatized than yourself, the golden rules are:

* be an active listener - open your heart and your mind to what is being said by the injured;

* don't give false reassurances or be insincere i.e. don't lie, but always be tactful and diplomatic when you tell a truth; and

* don't exaggerate the situation or become emotional yourself. The person receiving first aid is already traumatized – don't add to it and certainly, don't lean on the traumatized one for your emotional support. Yes, they're strong, but give them a fair go!

For every traumatic event, everything that happens or is decided afterwards will be in context to the *nature* of the traumatic event – whether it's catastrophic, life-threatening, a repeat of previous similar events, happening to someone else rather than you, involves multiple people, involves death, and so on.

How you answer the D and R questions will help you to plan a way forward from that initial point of impact, and also play a large part in your emotional recovery going forward.

You may already know yourself well enough to be able to evaluate how well you responded to and recovered from a past event. But for some of you, the mere act of going over memories now, reflecting on your past trauma(s), will help you to gain a greater awareness of yourself and how you responded at that point in time.

For many people the initial impact of a traumatic event may only produce mild emotional responses but, for others the symptoms can be more severe, and the potential for prolonged symptoms is heightened. No-one knows immediately after an event has passed whether they will still be responding to or reliving that event next week, next month, next year or even years into the future. The event itself, and the imagery involved, is all that can usually be taken in at the time.

At the time of the events in my past, my thoughts never turned to "gosh, how will I feel about this later?" And I would doubt that anyone who is surviving through a traumatic event is thinking about anything other than what's happening in the moment. They'll likely think about others or their future after the initial shock is over, but at the time of the event thinking more laterally and exploratively is usually not how the conscious mind works in a fight-or-flight situation. In that instant the event occurs, the mind is usually only focused on determining the best course of action for one's own and immediate survival. And, given that traumatic events are usually unplanned, uncontrolled and extreme, there is usually no rationalization of 'futures' at the immediate time of impact. You're in the moment, it's in your face, and you're dealing with it *right then and there.*

For an event that is lengthy, such as the Thredbo Landslide and rescue operation, or a battle in war or a natural disaster, there will be times during the event's entirety where you will likely reflect on what's happened and possibly think of the future. For many people thinking 'futures' at that point, after the initial shock is over as mentioned before, is a natural thing to do and part of their inbuilt survival response (i.e. when we focus on the future we 'see' a future and that automatically supports the likelihood of survival). The mind will wander and feelings will fluctuate as they need to during and immediately after an event, and remembering that what you have experienced is a '*normal response to an abnormal situation*' is the key thing.

Further, it's the very personal nature of trauma that makes it so challenging to rationalize, even later on. Rationalizing something is usually helped along by having something else to compare it to, some reference point. With most traumatic events, unless they're the repetitive kind (in which case you *do* have those reference points and comparisons readily at hand), there's less of a likelihood that you'll immediately make sense of what's happened. Your only reference point is yourself and how *you* feel. For example, you might think to yourself "this hasn't happened to me before.......What do I do? How do I handle it?"

That's partly why literature on coping with a major personal crisis, such as that distributed by organizations like the Red Cross, always emphasizes that what you have experienced "is a unique and personal event"[xxxvi] and that there are specific steps you can take and pitfalls to avoid, to allow normal healing to take place.

****

Generally speaking, a person's response to a traumatic event can include any of the following **normal responses to the abnormal situation**:

- shock, including about what happened, who or what caused the event
- disbelief, including a "why me?" attitude or questioning the senselessness or injustice of the event
- viewing the event as surreal (like a movie or a dream)
- feelings of guilt or self-blame (e.g. survivor's guilt, or for not preventing the event), tension, sadness, terror, horror, shame, frustration, anxiousness, irritability, depression, hostility/unfriendliness/anger, numbness (i.e. emotions being cut off), fear (e.g. of a recurrence, of losing control again), of being let-down, disappointment, and/or of euphoria (i.e. a joy of survival, feeling high or excited and strong)
- a sense of longing, for all that has gone and will not be again
- helplessness, given that crises can reveal human frailties as well as strengths
- rapid mood changes
- significantly impaired concentration
- confusion
- forgetfulness
- tiredness
- dizziness
- palpitations
- the shakes
- difficulty breathing
- lowered self-efficacy
- sleep disturbances (e.g. insomnia, nightmares)
- an exaggerated startle reflex (i.e. easily startled)
- psychosomatic responses (including chest, neck and back pain)

- altered behaviour including avoidance, social withdrawal, decreased intimacy, lowered trust in others, blaming others
- substance abuse (i.e. alcohol and other drugs)
- menstrual disorders, including a sense of dragging in the womb, noting that miscarriages can often occur after a traumatic event
- muscle tension
- headaches

These responses are common and normal. By our very human nature expressing our feelings doesn't mean that we are out of control or having a breakdown, and even intense feelings usually only occur for limited periods.

An acute stress reaction is most often experienced when there has been a psychic injury, and a psychic injury can often accompany or be a consequence of a physical injury. This is particularly so when the trauma has resulted from an accident, some form of assault, a natural disaster, community violence or war.

Children experience an acute stress reaction in a similar way to adults, however the severity of their responses is closely related to whether or not they are separated from their family members or the event involves their family. Further, their recovery from the traumatic event is closely connected to the recovery of those who are responsible for caring for them.

Similarly an event can impact people much more intensely when more extreme conditions exist and often in relation to the following groups of people (who would be deemed at higher risk of trauma):

- where the event has resulted in a death, particularly multiple, sudden or violent deaths; when a child or youth dies; when the body is not found; or when the relationship with the deceased was difficult;
- the elderly – this is a result of readjustment sometimes being harder or there being reduced energy or time to rebuild;

- those evacuated, hospitalized or isolated/alone – due to these folks losing the support of friends, family or community; or when isolation is due to language barriers or cultural differences;
- those who are unwell or performance challenged[xxxvii] (my preferred word in lieu of 'disabled') – given that these people may need special care and support;
- those for whom the event is in addition to other traumatic events or crises in their lives;
- people who exhibit a throwback response to a previous loss or trauma; and
- emergency workers, volunteers or first aiders/helpers – especially those who have given deeply of themselves; came into direct contact with the injured, dying or dead; felt they didn't do their jobs properly; or experienced 'burnout'.

Often-times people respond emotionally to a traumatic event in a cyclic way – expressing how they feel one time or putting feelings on hold at another time. The event and your feelings about it may return in your thoughts, daydreams, through mental images, night dreams, flashbacks and even nightmares. You may remember past events and crises too, however these are all normal ways for the mind and heart to process the event and make meaning of it. Blocking feelings when they become too painful, or pushing things out of their mind (suppressing memories as they come back from the subconscious) are not good strategies however, as this may lead to loss of concentration, mental fuzziness and exacerbation of other responses. The earlier you are able to face and deal with your feelings, the sooner your healing will begin. Prolonging your emotional response to a traumatic event and perpetuating bad feelings and thoughts, and therefore avoiding the inevitable, shouldn't ever be a conscious decision that you make. The more you consciously block yourself from healing, the more difficulties later.

When there have been sustained or repeat traumatic events, or where initial post-trauma symptoms have not abated to any noticeable degree and the emotional responses become chronic, this is most often when we see one or more of the following post-traumatic stress symptoms prevail: substance abuse, depressive states, intrusive thoughts, prolonged feelings of fear and/or anxiousness, a strong push to take control of everything in one's life, social withdrawal, and/or prolonged sleep disturbances (e.g. chronic insomnia, the same recurring nightmares).

However, in whichever context the symptoms are presenting – immediate or prolonged – paying attention to the multifaceted and subjective aspects are critical to appreciating that the traumatic events invoke a range of different emotional responses in people. Some people may experience only one kind of response, some all of them. Each individual who's been injured by the event must therefore be viewed and respected (for their inherent rights to achieve a full recovery) both holistically and individually, and their recovery and rehabilitation managed accordingly.

Equally important is for you to view and acknowledge your personal experiences with trauma, rather than compare yourself to others. While it's useful to know how other people have responded to trauma, there's nothing to be gained (and potentially a whole lot of angst or conflict to be created) by comparing post-trauma symptoms, applying a value judgement as to which symptom is worse than another, or even questioning your own emotional response(s) to a traumatic event.

When your mind processes the traumatic event, some of the imagery will create memories, whereas some images may well be immediately forgotten. The subconscious (or unconscious) mind is where your memories are stored – a bit like a filing cabinet ready for easy retrieval of useful information – and it's important to understand that memories will exist until such time as the mind no longer needs them.

With the exception of some catastrophic illnesses and neurological conditions which deprive a person of their capacity for effective memory recall or the actual memories themselves are lost as a consequence of the physical brain deteriorating, human survival dictates the need for memories to exist or not. Memories are there either to ensure our happiness or our protection against future threat. Without memories, the archives of all our experiences, we would not have any way of making informed decisions, even at the basic of levels.

Risk management is something that happens in our lives every day. Each day we see things, make a value judgment what to do and what not to do. Memories are essential to the risk assessment step (of analyzing and evaluating) and the judgment(s) we make lead to our decision about how best to treat the risk(s). Therefore, without memories to reference and enable discernment to occur, effective risk management becomes almost impossible. Is it any wonder then that dementia sufferers, for example, are so at risk?

Even though some of your memories of a traumatic event may be not-so-nice, honouring your memories while you still have them (rather than seeing them as the enemy within) is going to be an enormous help when it comes time for you to let go of the pain associated with the memories. From my own experience I know, without doubt, that it was the emotional pain I was holding onto, associated with the memories of my various traumas, that complicated things for me quite unnecessarily. It wasn't the memories themselves that were the issue. In Chapter 5 I explore more about the need to validate and apply the relevance test to your memories when you're emotional responses have become chronic and begun adversely impacting your life.

In *No Boxing Allowed* I've also dedicated some sections to explaining how the mind works, how memories are filtered and retrieved, how pain associated with memories can create debilitating emotional 'baggage', how emotional baggage can be removed, as well as how to grow beyond fear. Emotionally letting go, what I refer to as emotional exfoliation[xxxviii], is one of the pivotal things to do and I explore this more in Chapters 5 and 6.

Enduring and surviving a traumatic event is enough on its own. But taking some time later, to focus on understanding your own emotional responses, and how the experience has changed you and your life, is going to be a great advantage to you in the long run. It will definitely enhance your capacity to endure and develop resilience.

When you place focus on someone else before you have healed yourself, you're pushing that useful, helpful energy away from your own being. No doubt others may benefit from your selfless approach, however at some point being attentive to yourself *first* is going to be far more beneficial to your immediate and longer term recovery. I always advocate for selflessness as the best posture to adopt in life, under normal life conditions, however in terms of you needing time to heal yourself after trauma, being a little less selfless for a while is going to be a good thing.

The experiential learning gained from a traumatic event is, as I mentioned earlier, a very personal and therefore subjective thing. Learning the 'theory' or science about something is all well and good as a *starting* point to understanding how and why events occur, or a way to go back and evaluate an experience, however experiential learning and being in the moment is, without a doubt, the more impressionable of the two methods of learning.

When you hear the term "street smart" or "the school of hard knocks" I'd guess that you'd know straight away what they mean. Perhaps if you could look at life post-trauma in terms of you being "trauma smart", this might help you realize the 'advantages' that can be gained from your experiences.

When all said and done, the reality is that we cannot erase the past. Whether the traumatic event was something you did or didn't cause or contribute to, or whether it was something you witnessed, it is still an event in the past.

That said, most things we experience in our lives are still worthy of our reflection, noting any lessons learned and then *applying* the learnings, as this is what will contribute most profoundly to your growth in life and help improve your ability to the empathetic towards and compassionate with others. Learning lessons from experience is great but, remember, if you don't *apply the learnings* and *see the results of that application*, the wisdom will never come.

****

I haven't referred much to the timing of traumatic events, e.g. whether they occurred years ago or more recently, so I want to take some time now to look at how what happens to us in our a formative years and our upbringing, influences who we become and how we manage things later in life.

In 1998 it was reported ^{xxxix} that British scientists had discovered that the human pain threshold is not inherited, but more likely influenced by upbringing. The press article quotes from Germany's *Psychologie Heute* magazine, a piece written by director of twin research at St Thomas' Hospital in London: "A person's pain threshold is determined much more strongly through contact with family and close friends than through genetic make-up". The testing regime, using 600 sets of twins, consisted of both identical (genetically identical) sets of twins and non-identical (genetically different) sets of twins. Approximately half and half.

As part of the study the scientists subjected the twins to steadily rising pressure on the forehead and the test subjects were asked to report when they felt the first sensation of pain. In all cases, both twins in a pair responded at approximately the same time. The scientists believe, therefore, that this "rules out genetic similarity as the reason for a similar sensation of pain. Upbringing, they said, was the crucial factor, including the way in which parents reacted to their own and their children's pain".

Some children certainly appear to be resilient, often times more than adults, however the impact of a traumatic event on them should never be underestimated in its intensity. Firstly because children generally have less experiences to fall back on than adults (fewer reference memories), and secondly because their processing of memories will be done without the need to necessarily create emotional baggage (i.e. children become happy again after trauma much more quickly than most adults do).

It's also generally understood that the younger the human the more flexible their capacity to heal and the faster their rate of healing. This is reflected most clearly in the fact that our body's and bodily functions change, and metabolic processes usually slow down, as we age. A two year who's undergone a major operation will usually heal much more quickly than an adult having the same operation.

I remember having to have my tonsils out (at age 19) when they were found to be nigh-on-useless in doing their job. The doctors made clear to me that my surgery would have been far less risky and my recovery far easier if I'd been under the age of 10. I found out post-op that the doctors were right, having gone through a range of post-op complications including losing a life-threatening volume of blood immediately after surgery. Within weeks though I was back to normal and the event didn't leave any lasting emotional or physical effects, but I learned the lesson from that surgery and applied the learnings when I had my own child to take care of, and make care decisions for.

A child's speed of healing is also reflected in the fact that children are far less rigid in their thinking than adults. As you age, and gain all those memories that help you be happy and survive, you may (though not always) become quite fixed or set in your thinking about how things should be done, how you should react/respond, how people should help you, and so on. It is the very nature of the mind-body connection that can actually get you into trouble later in life, and especially so if you've endured multiple traumatic events over many years, or repeat traumatic events. How quickly you bounce back from trauma will depend significantly on how fixed your thinking (and action) becomes over time. The more flexible and adaptable you are, the faster you will heal. The more rigid and inflexible (and stubborn) you are, the longer and potentially more painful the healing process.

At a societal level though, what we are seeing in the 21st Century is a far greater frequency of violent incidents, gun crime, hate crime and bullying. Throughout history, both modern and ancient, violence between humans has (unfortunately) always existed. It's one of the choices people make that, quite frankly, I will *never* understand, but nonetheless it's real.

The difference this century though, is that *children* are being subjected to far more violence and witnessing extreme events more so than any other time in our history. In a very recent article published in the USA by ABC News[xl], recognition is given to the fact that in some US communities "violence is a traumatizing part of everyday life" and that what is underappreciated "is the long-term psychological effects this sort of exposure to violence can have on children".

The article quotes from Chicago statistics on murder and shootings, highlighting the incredulous facts:

- during 2016, 762 murders and 4,367 shootings occurred – an average of 2 murders and 12 shootings per day, all year long!

- nine children under the age of 15 years have been killed during the period January 1ˢᵗ to the date of article (41 days) – that's an average of 1 child killed every 4.5 days! If that rate of killing were to continue, around 81 children under 15 years of age will die *just in Chicago during 2017*!

The article then goes on to quote another researcher who "explains what life is like for many kids who have been exposed to deadly violence:

That shaken sense of safety can lead to a wide array of symptoms............

They may be struggling with distressing memories of what happened, such as having nightmares and flashbacks, and this can make it difficult to concentrate and pay attention..........They can experience hyper-arousal, which is when you are more likely to have a startled response or be very frightened in situations where you are not necessarily facing the same threat, but you feel like that same threat is there." "Other symptoms include trouble eating and sleeping and experiencing aches and pains that aren't related to an acute illness."

The article further explains that a report from Chicago's Cook County Hospital cited more than 40% of (gun violence) patients screened showed signs of post-traumatic stress, and summarizes with the statement "That is a lot of pain and suffering." The article concludes with the revelation that poor communities, where high rates of gun violence tend to prevail, are not able to access the right kind of support services they need. This situation ultimately means the children in these neighbourhoods are the most vulnerable of all.

How so many children, and adults, survive day-in-and-day-out when they are surrounded by gun violence, war, communities displaced, or become refugees on the run from same, is nothing short of a miracle. If you are one of those survivors, I commend you for your courage and determination against the greatest adversity.

And out of respect for your experiences, I do not claim to know what that kind of trauma is like to endure because I've never lived it. Or someone who's fought in a war, been captured or tortured, injured or seen battle deaths? So too do I not claim to know what that kind of trauma is like to endure, because I have never experienced that either. BUT, and it's a huge BUT, one trauma is no less significant than another, as the person on the receiving end of the trauma is the *only one* who has true context and reference.

I don't know what your own personal experience with trauma is, however I want to assure you that if you are a survivor of childhood trauma that event has definitely contributed in at least one positive way to who you are today as an adult. Likewise the environment in which you were raised and the 'health' of the family unit in which you lived, have all contributed to who you are today as an adult.

Something about what you went through, what you saw happen or not happen (that should have), how others were with you, would have resulted in some sort of positive outcome. When you take a moment to reflect on your past, and compare that to you in the now, some examples of positive outcomes that come from experiencing trauma are things like:

* the gaining of insight, improved self-awareness, or improved understanding of others;

* an appreciation of life risk(s), an understanding of human behaviour, or an understanding of the importance of love and caring for others;

* knowing your pain threshold, developing strength of mind, or learning how to be tenacious in the face of adversity and resistance.

All the foundational traits and self-esteem building that as an adult you may well be overlooking or taking for granted, could well have come (and probably did come) from your childhood experiences.

****

The last aspect of experience with trauma that I think needs exploration is the trauma 'environment' – the context of the traumatic event and the direct relationship to your life, be it social or work related, and your level of control over that environment.

I spoke a little above about war and violence-ravaged communities and, together with acts of terrorism, these are probably the most prominent of traumatic events that we see and hear about every day in the news. Beyond them, vehicle and transportation accidents, domestic violence, school and community shootings, police interventions, peacekeeping activities, rebuilding of war torn communities, and human trafficking come a close second in being newsworthy. However, for whatever reason, what we don't hear much about (still) are the workplace traumatic events that leave families devastated.

Except for military personnel fighting battles and wars (which are uncontrolled spaces where the worker and employer have an entirely different set of risk management practices to put in place), injuries arising from workplace or work-related traumatic events are no less important than injuries arising from environmental, family or community-based events. Trauma to an individual is just that, trauma, and it doesn't matter where the event occurs or the context of the event, the traumatic event has resulted in injury to the individual(s) involved and also taken away any real semblance of control.

A couple of years ago, The Washington Post published an article about Sebastian Junger [xli] , "the much-celebrated war correspondent who spent months in combat with U.S. soldiers in Afghanistan.........(who) coped with post-traumatic stress that left him panicking in a New York subway station, "absolutely convinced I was going to die."" Junger recounted being on a front-line position that had just been taken from the Taliban, including the Taliban's counterattack which started with an hour-long rocket barrage, and how all he and others could do was curl up in the trenches and hope. Junger stated "I felt deranged for days afterwards, as if I'd lived through the end of the world." Junger was suffering an acute stress reaction.

Regarding the subway incident, Junger wrote that "There were too many people on the platform, the trains were coming into the station too fast, the lights were too bright, the world was too loud.......(and)... I was far more scared than I'd ever been in Afghanistan."

Whilst he had always written about the horrors that the military were facing, and was well known for that support, Junger went on from this traumatic time to suggest several ways for combat troops to be reintegrated back into American society, including allowing veterans of war to be able to speak in public about their experiences.

Junger's rationale was that he was seeing societies being disassembled over many generations, as a result of spiritual cannibalization. His notion about how we can really save veterans, was founded in societies looking at how to save themselves. He said "If we do that, the vets will be fine. If we don't, it won't matter anyway." Junger is right. Societies have to help themselves.

However, whilst Junger's experience is not an isolated one, neither should it be excluded from consideration here as a 'workplace' event. The fine line between what Junger experienced and what military personnel experienced, is only limited by the actual role each of those people played in the battlefield.

Junger may have been carrying a weapon for protection and/or to use against the 'enemy', however that was not his first "job". His workplace at the time was a war zone, yes, however it was a completely unregulated and uncontrolled workplace where his actual employer would have (quite rightly) defaulted to the military, to allow them to make that battlefield as 'safe' as possible for Junger to be there. However, the military personnel who were his colleagues in the battlefield, *did* have the "job" of fighting and their workplace, in that context, was not one that any of them, or their employer, could control.

A traumatic event that occurs in any work or social context is likely to involve other people, is not going to follow a pattern, and the environment is probably not going to be one that you can readily control yourself. Your capacity to influence how an event is managed is directly relative to the environment in which the event has occurred. For instance, if the event happens at a school the management of it will be different to if the event happened in a home.

In a school communication protocols, evacuation plans and emergency response procedures normally exist to manage an event and its aftermath. The environment is known to you, but not to as intimate a level as some other environments.

In a home, especially if it's your home, you're more likely to have a greater awareness of how to manage the risks that result from an event because you know the environment well, perhaps intimately.

In a workplace the communication protocols, evacuation plans and emergency response procedures will be in place (and often times rehearsed) and whilst this environment is known to you because you would only spend about 1/3 of your day there your level of awareness of the environment will be lower than for other more well-known places, like in your own home or a friend's home.

Recovery and healing for trauma survivors (including through formal or informal rehabilitation programs) is therefore going to be a unique experience, and will be influenced by the environment in which the event took place. Where there are third parties with a legal obligation to protect you, involved in your recovery and rehabilitation, then the way your rehabilitation is managed may well be very different than if you called all the shots. This 'third party' involvement scenario is particularly relevant when an employer, or community entity, has legal obligations to manage the emergency aspects of the traumatic event, or where you are the employee and subject to an employer's rehabilitation policy and procedures.

A simple thing to remember is that as each type of environment presents its own risks and event scenarios, so too the difference in environmental context can act to help you differentiate causal factors, and rationalize the event after it is over. Environment provides you with a personal context for the trauma you endure, but it doesn't define who you are, what after-effects you will experience, or how well you will recover.

CHAPTER 4

Making choices for your recovery and healing, including when to say "when"

Probably the single most important aspect of this chapter is the importance of a positive self-fulfilling prophecy.

A self-fulfilling prophecy is a prediction that directly or indirectly causes itself to become true, by the very terms of the prophecy itself, due to positive feedback between belief and behavior (actions).

If your prophecy (i.e. prediction or forecast) about the future and healing from a traumatic event is bleak, then your outcome is most likely going to be bleak. If your prophecy is positive and empowering, and you are steadfast in maintaining a positive vision of who you want to be at the end of the recovery and healing period, then your actions will match your beliefs. A positive outcome becomes your self-fulfilling prophecy.

The true power behind a self-fulfilling prophecy is always the individual. It doesn't matter one iota what anyone else thinks or does, if you believe it yourself and the outcome you want is within the realm of possibilities (taking into account all the factors of the traumatic event, the injury/ies you sustained, and the after-effects you may still be experiencing), then your prophecy will hold true.

There is nothing so powerful than the visioning of a positive outcome, even against all the obstacles and barriers placed in your way, and the ultimate fulfilment of that outcome. But the most important factor is *your level of emotional recovery and healing from a traumatic event is yours to determine, not someone else's to dictate*.

If your injury was a physical one, then there may well be real limitations to how well you can recover and heal. There's no point ignoring facts, but visualizing a best-case scenario in the physical realm (within the real limitations that exist) is better than giving in and giving up. You can't suddenly put back a limb, but you could acquire an artificial limb that can give you back freedom and mobility. You can't suddenly grow a new internal organ, but you may be able to receive a transplant or use medical means or medications to give you back some of that lost functionality. Ultimately though, looking beyond the limitations set by established medical models is critical.

When Christopher Reeve had his riding accident and landed himself on a respirator and in a wheelchair, not once did he lose sight of what could be and not once did he refuse to work through the barriers placed in front of him by 'modern medical science'. He advocated for new research into spinal injuries, he had a go at everything that *he felt comfortable would help him*. Christopher made the decisions, on advice where relevant, and *he led* his efforts to live as full and complete a life as possible, despite his catastrophic physical injuries.

What psychic injuries he sustained as a result of that horse riding event or what followed are not widely known, however his mental and emotional resilience was clearly demonstrated in his own decision making about his physical injuries, his years of fighting against the adversities he faced, and the fact that he remained as helpful, pleasant, selfless and joyful as possible throughout his entire life post-accident.

Christopher Reeves' life and how he coped with his major personal crisis is testament to a human's capacity and willpower. Like so many hundreds of thousands, if not millions, of people who have endured traumatic events and gone on to build lives of purpose and positivity, his legacy lies in the power of the mind and the heart to see his emotional recovery achieved. Full healing from a physical injury may not always be possible, and this can leave scars at an emotional level too, but the mere act of recovering and healing at an emotional level is going to add many-fold to improving how you manage life within any physical limitations you may be experiencing.

If the only injury you suffered was a psychic one, then you (and only you) can and should take full control over how your mind thinks and how your heart feels in response to that injury. Even your immediate emotional response to a traumatic event, whether or not you sustain an actual psychic *injury* from the event, is yours to own. No-one else makes you feel or think a certain way, or is responsible for how you feel or think.

An emotional response to something is as unique as the person is unique. No two people will respond exactly the same way to an event and therefore *how* people are helped with their immediate emotional response or to heal from the psychic injury/ies sustained during the event, must be done in context to the person and the dynamics of their life.

The not-so-funny part about injuries at an emotional level is that, like with a lot of physical injuries, the observers of the injured person tend to be the 'experts' in what is best to help the injured person recover and heal. Where a physical injury can be so severe it clearly indicates that full healing is not likely to ever be achieved – an amputation of a limb is a perfect example – the support for the injured usually follows a certain path and the injury remains easily discernible by the observer and the injured. However the often-times silent, psychic injuries aren't always as discernible or noticeable.

Under a standard medical model, effective injury management of the psychic injury can be inadvertently pushed down in the list of treatment and recovery priorities and, in some cases, even go unnoticed or ignored. Also, the injured person may see their own psychic injury as not as important as the physical injury when, in reality, both kinds of injuries are just as important as one another.

Conversely, under a mental health model the mental health aspects are almost too much in the forefront and the link between body and mind often-times gets ignored. The focus is all about symptom management - controlling, treating and (hopefully) relieving symptoms - rather than addressing root causes and removing symptoms altogether. *Managing* something is completely different to *eliminating* something – the end result is not the same. In managing symptoms the symptoms perpetuate; in eliminating symptoms, they no long exist.

It is only through looking at root causes, and *acknowledging that what happened actually caused the psychic injury in the first place*, that your symptoms can be understood. When symptoms and their root causes are fully understood and rationalized, that's when they can start to reduce in intensity and, over time, be successfully removed altogether. At the point when your symptoms disappear, that's when your recovery and healing from the psychic injury will be complete.

If you allow yourself to believe that there was something already inside you that caused the psychic injury to occur, or allow other people to insinuate that it was because of some kind of insecurity, deficiency, or incapacity in you, then you will have immediately placed yourself in the passenger (and victim) seat, not the driver's seat. **The event caused the injury to you; you didn't cause the injury to yourself.** The notion that some people have a tendency to suffer emotional injury ahead of others is ignoring the very fact that people experience **a normal response to an abnormal situation.**

In any effective incident (and injury) investigation process the key things an investigator looks for are:

- location, context, consequences/outcomes of the incident;
- the likelihood of the incident occurring again;
- type/nature, extent/severity and bodily location of injuries, and which are primary and secondary;

- the 'mechanism' of injury – how it happened i.e. the method of injury (e.g. falling from height, being hit by a car, being crushed, assault by another person);
- the 'agent' of injury – what caused the injury i.e. the source of energy, such as a physical object (metal bar, gun, piece of equipment, machine etc.), animal, another person, environmental factor (temperature, noise, vibration, storm etc.), chemical, biological factor, and so on.

When an employer puts in place preventative measures to improve health and safety for employees and visitors to their workplaces, the golden key to preventing future incidents (and therefore minimizing future injuries or deaths), is effectively risk managing the *mechanisms and agents* of injury as their highest priority. Australian Standard (AS) 1885.1 is a sound reference document for employers in Australia (and elsewhere) to help them prevent and manage outcomes from workplace incidents that result in injury or disease. In fact, I wish more people knew about this standard and applied it in their everyday lives, as risk management of incidents occurs in every context not just work, and prevention is always far better than cure.

Any effective, best practice prevention program (for health and safety management, or a rehabilitation program for return-to-work or return-to-home) will always factor root cause analysis in somewhere. In rehabilitation terms the root cause analysis should be done during the Self-Assessment or Initial Needs Analysis (INA) stage. Sometimes an injured person can't do their own Self-Assessment in which case an external INA is normally done by a certified and accredited rehabilitation provider and the findings used to inform treatments/therapies, medical interventions, and any transitioning steps such as a graduated return to work/home.

Root cause analysis is an investigatory process that looks to uncover hidden or previously unknown factors that have contributed to an event, the injury/ies and other repercussions resulting from the event, and the people or processes in place at the time of the event. The most effective root cause analysis is done by working backwards from the event and injury itself, from the signs and symptoms that are presenting in the 'present', to the actions, inactions, signs and symptoms that occurred or didn't occur in the 'past'. Root cause analysis involves asking clarification questions along the way, until all the data that could possibly be acquired is there, ready for analysis of the linkages, interdependencies, duplicities, and irrelevancies (i.e. things that are identified as part of the data gathering exercise, but later found not to be contributing factors to either the event or the injury/ies). And, when root cause analysis is done impartially (without unfair judgement, emotion or bias applied) then the outcomes will remain robust and informative for the future.

Fundamentally, if you don't know why and how you got hurt, and by what, then you can't fully understand context and rationalize the injury, and determine how to heal from it later on. Root cause analysis can be done by you at any time, in any context and as often as you want. In fact, root cause analysis is really a foundation stone for living a sound life, where risks are managed effectively and in context to your life, and where your decisions are made with discernment and maturity, rather than from an emotive or rushed base.

****

In the vein of prevention being better than cure, I want to take a moment to look at strategies for achieving good mental and emotional health and preventing psychic injury.

The three main goals in relation to good mental and emotional health can be summarized as (i) know yourself well – your strengths, limitations, and deficiencies – and treat yourself well, (ii) prevent injury to yourself wherever possible, and (iii) if injury does occur, analyze the issues and challenges that you face including the root causes of your injury and symptoms.

Achieving and maintaining good mental and emotional health depends on a range of things, not the least being your diet. Eating well, balancing nutritious food and water and minimizing alcohol and other drugs (including smoking), will boost your immune system and improve your resistance to mental dysfunction and emotional imbalance. Likewise remaining active and exercising regularly, in proportion to your age, works immediately to improve both mental and emotional wellbeing as well as overall body functioning – e.g. metabolic rate, cardiovascular function, muscle tone, and endorphin and serotonin release. Building healthy and happy relationships with others, as well as thinking good thoughts about yourself, all work to create a sense of 'goodness' prevailing in your life.

Taking control of your future is pivotal to achieving the goals that you set and having a sense of purpose. And, when you hold yourself fully accountable for your own success in life, even against the worst adversities, and not use other people or a situation as an excuse to play the victim card or apply blame, then you are immediately empowering yourself for a positive outcome – this is where the self-fulfilling prophecy well and truly come to the fore!

At this point you're probably thinking to yourself "how on earth do I know what the root causes of my post-trauma symptoms are?" I know from personal experience, that it takes a considerable focus on 'inner' self and feelings, and accepting the memories arising from an event, in order to get to the truth and even *begin* to understand yourself well enough to tackle the symptoms head on. The next chapter has more about this. What we'll do here first, is look at aspects of recovery using a timeline or step-by-step approach, and hopefully this will help you to see the path of best choice for you; from the event itself, right through all the stages of your life post-event.

Helping yourself, staying in control of the course of actions and remaining true (in your mind and heart) to the prophecy you have set, through all stages of recovery and healing, is first and foremost. Holding a positive mindset where you're helping yourself first, and staying self-motivated, is not only your *foundation for the future*, but also the *umbrella strategy* under which all the steps going forward will be included. There's no point making a decision about actions unless you've first determined your strategy, as the strategy addresses and summarizes '*why*' you're choosing to do something. The decisions to be made (e.g. formal rehabilitation plan, combining medical treatments with meditation sessions, alternative therapies, etc.) address and summarize the '*what*' and, lastly, your actions/to-do list summarizes '*how*' the decisions will come to life.

When you look at your recovery and healing from trauma no differently than you would any other outcome in life, e.g. moving house, building a new house, paying off your mortgage, gaining a qualification, or even applying for a new job, then it can be broken down into those three key elements (why, what, how) and managed in realistic chunks.

Furthermore it's really important that you stay focused on doing for yourself and developing self-reliance. Whilst it's perfectly OK to accept and receive essential help from others when it's needed, to become reliant on others when you can actually do those things for yourself, is going to hinder your capacity to develop resilience in the face of adversity and potentially kill any self-motivation traits that you may have already developed. At no time should you complain about what you're not receiving from others, until you've done *everything* you can to help yourself.

When you're in 'help myself' mode a natural inclination can often be to gather all the information you can get your hands on. Mothers-to-be sometimes do this when they're preparing for the birth of their first baby - reading book after book, researching on the WWW, asking friends and family about their stories. As a consequence information overload can happen, stressors can be introduced unnecessarily, and anxiety or overprotectiveness of self can result.

One of the key things about information gathering is learning when too much is too much, or when enough is enough. If you start your recovery and healing journey with too much information, finding the tree in the forest will be challenging, if not impossible. Start small and simple, remember my version of KISS, and build on the information you need, or discard stuff that's no longer needed as you journey along. Remember, you're in control all the way.

Fundamental to keeping it simple is to forget the labels and restrictions others place on or around you. Saying to yourself "I got hurt and I want to get better" is the level of simplicity I'm talking about here. Focus on the core issue, not the white noise.

Just because the observers are wanting to diagnose you doesn't mean you have to agree with their diagnosis, or adopt the treatment regime they are imposing on you. In the case of best practice, formalized rehabilitation programs these focus all parties, especially the rehabilitee, on a structured, informed and well-paced rehabilitation program that has specific and agreed goals for all to achieve. These best practice rehabilitation programs *always* allow for the rehabilitee to make and own all the decisions about their care and, at an agreed point in time, 'take it from here'.

Any rehabilitation program that has an end goal of labelling the rehabilitee as permanently disabled, or involves an enduring regime of treatment (be it drugs, invasive therapies, medical interventions or medical consultations) without any focus on determining root causes (to enable the root causes to be addressed and fixed within the rehabilitation program), is serving every stakeholder *except* the rehabilitee.

A perfect example of taking away control from the injured is illustrated in a 2015 article on Vietnam War veterans[xlii] which states that a new study revealed that "More than 40 years after fighting in Vietnam, about 11 per cent of combat veterans still suffer from post-traumatic stress disorder...... and far more of them are getting worse than are getting better". Whilst the article refers to the study's findings that "most people who serve in war are resilient" and that only a minority of those veterans develop post-traumatic stress, it clearly states that the study makes the claim that "if they're going to recover, they're going to recover early on".

The study appears to be one based on a mental health (including psychiatry) model, linked to Army research on the rate of diagnosis of a 'disorder', and is published by the American Medical Association. Further it is based on "2,348 Vietnam-era veterans" who, it appears, had either been formally diagnosed with and medically treated for post-traumatic stress, or were questioned about post-traumatic stress symptoms and whether, over time, they still experienced those symptoms or not.

Where the study draws the conclusion about 'early recovery or no recovery' this is, in my opinion, beyond ridiculous and arrogant. Therefore my response to both the article and the study, in terms of an individual's recovery timeline and prognosis, has to be "poppy cock". These are exactly the kinds of 'studies' that end up preventing or discouraging positive change in attitudes, beliefs, rehabilitation programs, medical interventions, treatment and/or recovery regimes. And they are the kinds of 'studies' that keep trauma survivors labelled, victimized, belittled, ignored and/or relegated to being disabled-for-life, when all of that is simply not in sync with how the human body works to heal itself, and how the mind and heart can be programmed to achieve a positive result, not a negative one. These 'studies' in fact create and promote a negative prophecy, not a positive one.

A further perfect example comes from the 1964 collision between the ships HMAS Voyager and HMAS Melbourne (Australian Navy ships) and the May 2004 update [xliii] that a compensation payment had been made to a sailor psychologically affected by experiencing the collision.

The occupational health and safety news article describes the event of February 1964 where HMAS Melbourne collided with HMAS Voyager around 9pm and cut it in two. Both sections of HMAS Voyager sunk within a few hours of each other, 82 lives were lost and many sailors in the stern section, which sunk last, were rescued from the water.

The 19 year old sailor who subsequently received the compensation payment of around $AU377,000 some 40 years later, was below deck at the time of the collision however, when he mustered on deck, he helped bring survivors and the deceased on board his ship. He also witnessed the stern section sinking and was concerned for the safety of one of his mates (buddies) on HMAS Voyager.

How damaged HMAS Melbourne was, was unknown by many, however when it arrived back in Sydney after the rescue operation had completed the sailors were instructed not to discuss the collision.

Almost 40 years after the event, the sailor sought to recover damages for psychological injury. His employer (possibly Australian Navy as the Commonwealth employer) admitted negligence and the Court only had to establish the fact that the sailor had in fact been psychologically injured and *experiencing the collision was what caused that injury*, for the claim for compensation to stand up.

The NSW Supreme Court accepted:

- what the sailor said he saw and experienced;
- that after the event the sailor had started to drink heavily;
- that about a year after the event the sailor began to have nightmares about drowning in the black sea; and
- that the dreams (nightmares) had remained with him since.

There were several witnesses called who attested to the change in the sailor's character.

Around 1998 the sailor had been required by the Commonwealth (Federal) government to attend examination, and the sailor was subsequently diagnosed with post-traumatic stress disorder (PTSD). He was referred to a PTSD program conducted by a hospital, attending from November through December 1999, and was prescribed anti-stress medication (for depression) and other medication for his sleeping issues. The article states "he had responded favourably and was in partial remission. However specialist medical opinion accepted by the Court indicated it was unlikely that there would be further significant improvement in his condition."

As another key factor "because of studies done in relation to World War I, World War II and Vietnam, the Court accepted the causal relationship between involvement of service personnel in traumatic events and the development of psychiatric disorders. Therefore it was not only foreseeable but likely that some of the sailors involved in the collision would suffer psychological injury. The sailor was entitled to damages."

Whilst I do not for one second question or judge the sailor for his symptoms, both immediate and prolonged, and I extend my empathy for him (knowing full well how debilitating ongoing nightmares can be), there are some key aspects to this story that I want to highlight, so that you can see the patterns, questions and issues that prevail:

> ** the sailors were instructed not to discuss the collision –* why is that? For security reasons, reputation management reasons, operational reasons? The employer better have had a bloody good reason for not letting these folks talk it out, and was that 'silence rule' ever investigated as a causal factor for the nightmares which started a year on from the event? Or the depression?

> How were these sailors expected to go about their normal lives without any kind of CISD or operational debriefing (in a group or individually)? Was root cause analysis ever entertained as an option or actioned, to bring to the surface all the issues and interdependencies?

> <u>My summary:</u> Nothing good will ever come when you prevent people from talking about something bad that has happened to them. By ordering silence after an event affected people are immediately forced to bottle things up and go it alone. That approach (as *un-strategic* as it actually is) is not at all conducive to recovery and healing.

> ** after the event the sailor had started to drink heavily –* the choices people make, especially the consumption of alcohol (which generally has an anesthetizing, depressive and/or sedative effect on the body), are ultimately *their choices*. No-one forces you to drink; you *choose* to drink. And the level of your consumption is a *choice* you make each time.

> Drinking (alcohol) can be a form of release or escape from reality, or a way to temporarily block feelings (because basically, if you drink too much your body feels numb and your mind ends up mimicking the body!). It is also viewed by many people as a way of enhancing or arousing their lives, when in fact it's achieving the exact opposite.

Drinking is known to cause a range of bodily responses, some benign by comparison to other social drugs, but nonetheless the body is always giving you signs that consumption should be well managed. The physiological impact of excessive or binge drinking can create anything from a permanent state of drunkenness, to worst case conditions like alcoholism, cirrhosis of the liver or alcohol-related-brain-damage (ARBD). ARBD is rarely talked about with any real focus being given to prevention or growing the database of morbidity and mortality data, even when there is already so much valid data (in community health settings) to support the root cause analysis of other diagnosed illnesses and diseases and their independencies with or linkages to ARBD.

Alcoholism has some classic symptoms:

- whole body responses - blackouts, dizziness, shaking, craving or sweating;
- behavioural and mood responses – aggression, agitation, compulsiveness, lack of restraint, self-destruction; anxiety, euphoria, discontent, loneliness, guilt;
- physical body responses – gastrointestinal reactions (nausea, vomiting), coordination issues or tremors, slurred speech.

However, what is well known in the field of natural therapies but not so commonly known by the medical profession (because they rarely look at emotional wellness when assessing a patient's health), is that drinking alcohol causes emotions to be suppressed for a time. If you can imagine an active volcano with a lid placed over the crater (at the top), at some point the contents (hot lava, rock, stream etc.) are going to want to escape, and violently.

Alcohol consumption (especially when excessive) by someone with unresolved emotional responses to past events or people, is no different to that volcano. *Before the alcohol,* things spew out bit by bit, there's regular rumbling but nothing that can't be managed by natural release mechanisms – a few hot emotional outbursts here and there, letting-off-steam - residual internal pressure keeps pushing things to the surface. But, once the alcohol is in your system, a bit like putting a lid over the crater, the emotional stuff gets pushed down and artificially suppressed. Pressure continues to build up inside, even though you feel euphoric and invincible. And when the effects of the alcohol wear off, or the pressure gets too much to cope with, that's when the big explosions happen – violent venting of anger, lashing out at people without discernment, self-harm, a flurry of nightmares, excessive fear responses, or 'clustering' of other symptoms like exaggerated startle reflexes.

My summary: The fact that there are other lifestyle choices in the sailor's life, and the employer made specific demands in relation to how the incident and its aftermath were managed, is directly relevant to understanding the sailor's symptoms and their causes.

Why did the sailor choose to drink (the inference being in the article that he was drinking to excess)? Did he have an earlier pattern of binge drinking? Did he already suffer from ARBD or alcoholism? Was it the event itself, the threat to his safety or his mates' safety, or his obvious lack of control over the event and its repercussions, which pivoted his choice to drink afterwards? To what extent did his drinking cause the nightmares or depression, or exacerbate a pre-existing condition, or create further symptoms that, collectively, could then be 'ticked off the list' as being so-called PTSD. I say so-called because, at this point in history, the D ('disorder') label given to post-traumatic stress is not proven in scientific terms. The term is only coined as a result of the gathering of anecdotal data that's based on individuals' perceptions of their symptoms. Further, disorder in itself deems a worst-case scenario outcome, rather than a positive outcome. You may recall I mentioned this in earlier chapters.

after the event the sailor was required to attend examination, was diagnosed with PTSD, attended a specific PTSD program for two months, was prescribed multiple medications for his symptoms, deemed in partial remission and unlikely to see improvement of his current condition – there is no mention of a formal and structured rehabilitation program that the sailor was consulted about and agreed to, so we cannot draw a conclusion either way. However, from the outcomes one can clearly see that the best case scenario did not play out for this sailor.

Why did he only attend a "program" for two months, when clearly his symptoms and the severity of the event suggest that a longer analysis of his injuries and his life (behaviours, tendencies, habits, inactions, physical and emotional status, and lifestyle choices), and a much longer period of recovery and healing, were all warranted?

Was the examination only done under a medical or mental health model, or was it done using a holistic whole-of-person model and include a physical examination and discussion of lifestyle and relationships? What other diagnoses resulted from his examination? Was he advised about his lifestyle choices? Was he offered less brain chemical-altering interventions (i.e. no medications) such as some form of life coaching, crisis counselling, or social skills development? Was his family/inner sanctum or employer advised or counselled in how to support him post-event? Was he given an opportunity to return to work in some capacity?

What form of follow up assessment or examination was done and at what intervals? Were other sailors (on board at the time of the event) assessed or examined in the same manner? What were their results? Surely this sailor wasn't the only one impacted by the traumatic event.

<u>My summary:</u> Looking at all the factors, researching all likely scenarios, doing root cause analysis of his symptoms would have helped build a more holistic and helpful picture for this sailor. For the 'system' to now see him as being in remission and likely never to fully recover is

automatically placing him in the too hard basket. As I explain in *No Boxing Allowed* "That basket, once created, will never get emptied.""[xliv]

****

As you can see there are so many factors to be considered when reflecting on past events and determining root causes. Its therefore no surprise that taking responsibility for your own recovery and healing after a traumatic event is going to be challenging and, for some, very daunting.

To get a handle on this from the outset, I recommend that you allow *time* to be on your side. Don't push yourself!

After a traumatic event, especially in those first days and weeks, there's a lot you can do to help yourself – help you to come to terms with the experience, reduce some of the stressors, and relieve any distress you may feel. Like with the D and R part of first aid, there are some simple yet effective and positive things you can do immediately after an event has happened and in the initial few weeks of your recovery:

* give yourself permission to feel rotten about what happened and what you went through, but stay focused on your strengths. Feeling angry is perfectly normal and will definitely help with the grieving process;

* be 'kind' to yourself;

* spend time with people you care about and who care about you;

* face reality – viewing a body, going to a funeral, revisiting the scene of the event, inspecting losses, or visiting other ill or injured – will all help you to come to terms with the event;

* look after yourself by eating well and regularly, getting plenty of rest and sleep, drinking lots of water, and maintaining regular exercise;

* reduce consumption of body-stimulating drinks like sodas, caffeinated coffees and teas, and greatly reduce or eliminate smoking and alcohol consumption. Your body is already going to feel a little hyper-aroused, so limiting or excluding stimulants is best;

* make time for relaxation such as listening to music, taking a bath, reading, going dancing or gentle walking – whatever works best for you and helps you to mentally and emotionally zone-out (the natural way);

* plan your days and schedule at least one meaningful activity each day. Don't be too rigid with the timetable, but make sure each day is balanced in the kinds of activities you do;

* hold off making big life decisions such as moving house or changing your job in the days and weeks following the event, however do make smaller decisions each day that give you back control over your life and outcomes;

* don't isolate yourself, but also take time to be alone with your own thoughts and feelings;

* stay informed about the event, if this is relevant, but remember to be on the lookout for information overload or rehashing things just for the sake of it. There will be no value in reinforcing the bad aspects, rather it will be more helpful to draw a line in the sand, acknowledge that you've been hurt, and then step over that line and walk forward;

* practice meditation or relaxation techniques when you feel strong emotions coming to the surface or that you are losing your sense of control. Pilates, yoga, ballet, tai chi, rowing and steady walking are very good physical exercise regimes to follow too, not just for general health but they also offer slow, deliberate and rhythmic actions which are helpful in helping the body to manage its response to stressors and bring about a sense of inner peace;

* be open to receiving support and comfort, and express your needs clearly and honestly to family, friends and others relevant;

* if children are involved, allow them to share with you and encourage them to express their own feelings. Allow them to return to school and keep up with their normal activities as soon as they are ready;

* don't bottle up your feelings or avoid talking. Whenever you want to, speak freely with trusted others about your experience and how it's affected you. Or if you don't want to do that, then write about it, like in a daily journal. Sharing pressure usually halves the pressure, but stay mindful that when you speak to others you should be attentive to what's going on in their lives and not become a "dumper" who dumps (rather than vents) all the negative on someone else[xlv]. Likewise, listen to others who've been affected by the event, and what they have to say about it and how they feel;

* drive more attentively/carefully and maintain usual safety standards;

* continue any routine medical treatments or other therapies. Stay in routine.

Going with the flow and valuing time as an 'enabler' of your recovery and healing, rather than seeing time as a test or an obstacle, is going to serve you better in maintaining a positive mindset.

Time is something that no-one can take from you after the event is over and, in most circumstances, time is actually going to be on your side at that point. After all, you survived the event!

In Stuart Diver's case, his rescue took the time that was necessary. Stuart couldn't influence how he was rescued or make it happen any quicker than it did, but once he was brought to the surface and given the immediate medical attention he needed, from that point on he was effectively in control. Time was on his side, even though time probably felt like it had stood still for those few days he was underground and trapped.

Stuart did receive emotional support while he waited under the rubble to be rescued, and there are media reports that he was supported during his recovery by volunteer counsellors as well. Ultimately though, his recovery post-event tracked over a timeline that he would have directly had control over, albeit with some influencing factors such as input from family/inner sanctum, the medical profession, counsellors, employer and/or friends.

Because a traumatic event momentarily takes away your control, once the event has passed it is essential that *you take control of your use of time from that point on*. Not only will that create an empowering and affirmative emotional response, giving you back the control you previously lost, it will also give you a chance to reflect, gather information, analyze root causes, rationalize, and decide your way forward.

If you are injured as a result of a work-related event, then hopefully you will have protection (through legislation or employer policies, or both) that allow you proper rehabilitation time and a structured return-to-work program (if that's what you agree to). If the traumatic event occurred somewhere else other than work, the same protections might apply (i.e. legislative protections, stakeholder legal obligations etc.) or you may be in a position to take the time that you need by having income-protection, health insurance or savings available.

For many folk though, the pressures and challenges of life are still going to be there even after an event is over and effective time management becomes even more important. Perhaps you'll have more on your plate to deal with after an event has passed - this will depend on the context of your life before and after the event, and who was and wasn't involved. Perhaps the traumatic event and injury/ies you sustained will add to your pressures and challenges, or reduce the time you have with family and friends.

Perhaps things will appear to speed up for you for a while. All these factors are things you need to consider, take control over, and not ignore.

Whichever way 'time' appears to track, the best mental approach you can take is to relax about in your head, and see time coupled with sound decision-making as taking care of what is best. We all know Mother Nature and time are good healers. Giving yourself time, even when others attempt to rob you of it, and putting your recovery and healing first on your personal to-do list (without being completely selfish in your approach), is the best complement to time.

Time is priceless[xlvi]. Don't squander it, but always see it as a free gift. When you value and harness time as an *enabler,* you will begin to see how it acts as a non-judgmental door that automatically opens up opportunities (and choices) for you in the future.

Holding yourself accountable and taking positive action when "when" comes. What this is about is knowing when your symptoms are adversely impacting your life and knowing that the time has come for you to take real control of your future and outcomes. No-one but you will know when you get to *that point,* when your acute post-trauma responses have turned into symptoms more consistent with post-traumatic stress, or are adversely impacting on your life and others around you.

While other people have no right or business telling you that your emotional responses are going to be around 'forever', *neither should you allow yourself to believe* in this kind of negative 'forever' scenario. The symptoms related to post-traumatic stress, or a prolonged emotional response to an event, are simply your body's way of telling you that something still hasn't settled down, that things haven't returned to the right level of balance yet and that your autonomic nervous system still reads that your body needs to be in fight or flight mode. Your body's GAS is working, but there's obviously a blockage (e.g. at the emotional level) somewhere, that's preventing true homeostasis (and balance) from being achieved.

In the world of natural therapies, the first thing we learn is that pain is the body's *last signal* to you that something is wrong. There may be a whole bunch of other signals of an injury (say like tingling, fear, heart palpitations, stomach upset, excessive body heat, headache, vision issues) that you may have ignored or brushed aside, however they are all the body's first signals to you that something is wrong.

If you ignore the first few rounds of signals, the body's loud and final wakeup call is going to be 'pain'. This can be physical pain, mental anguish and/or emotional pain. But, pain is pain and it should never be ignored.

Being fully accountable for your recovery and healing means running with the ball yourself. It doesn't mean hand-passing the decision-making ball to someone else. It's your life to live and you deserve to have control of important decisions - it's your inherent right. You shouldn't give away control over your health and life outcomes, anywhere or at any time.

In the next chapter I address recovery and healing from prolonged symptoms, including known post-traumatic stress symptoms, in the context of personal growth and improving self-awareness and we'll also explore some remedial actions you can take yourself to help you along that path. However in relation to accountability and realizing the turning points in life that we all face from time to time, it's important for you to acknowledge that at any point in life you are *free to choose* to recover and heal from the psychic injury/ies you've sustained, or remain a victim of circumstance. Deciding whether you will be the passenger or the driver of your life is likely the first major decision you will make during your recovery post-trauma. It is fundamental to the level of accountability you will hold yourself to deliver.

And remember, while you're fluctuating in indecision mode you are automatically not taking control. A bit like a fan that's running at full speed but the screw that's holding the blades in place is loose. The fan blades are still spinning but they're not in alignment and spinning smoothly.

I can understand a hesitancy to take control after a trauma – it's happened to me after some of the traumatic events I've survived. I was hurting so much inside I didn't 'know' *if or how* I could fix how I felt and the emotional responses that I was experiencing. After some events I was able to pick up the reins of control quickly and get back in the driver's seat, but after other events, the more extreme ones by comparison, the desire to pick up the reins was just not there, for a long time, and sometimes for what seemed like an eternity.

What you have to achieve is that level of 'knowing' - that you have a reset button inside yourself which you can press *at any time you choose*, when you reach the point of "when" with your post-traumatic stress symptoms.

From my own personal experience *I chose to fully heal* 20 years after the most significant traumatic event in my adult years. The event happened when I was 24, and I was not quite 45 years old when I finally made the choice that enough was enough. There were a number of external factors and other crises for me to manage which influenced how quickly I could get to the "when" point, but once I reached it there was no turning back. I took complete control of my life and health outcomes, made some major life (and change) decisions, and the result was nothing short of miraculous for my health and wellbeing.

Whilst I had never sought a diagnosis for the specific post-trauma symptoms I had experienced for that 20 some years, on and off, or had the need to be formally 'diagnosed' as suffering post-traumatic stress, my choice became all about my health and quality of life. It was as simple as me saying to myself "make a change or completely withdraw from the world". The first choice was ideal, the alternate was ridiculous. For me, healing at that time in my adult years also had nothing to do with the childhood traumatic events from which I had long healed, however it had *everything to do with when I was ready* - when I'd had enough of the symptoms and said "when" to myself.

For the medical profession to arrogantly claim, and program into the minds of people (using studies as 'proof') that a person has no capacity to recover and heal years, even decades, after an event has caused them a psychic injury, not only does that go against a doctor's own theoretical training in human physiology, it belies the GAS and the body's innate ability to heal itself when the right conditions exist to do so.

One of my greatest concerns in relation to the medical and mental health 'view' of post-traumatic stress is the pushing of psychiatric medications on injured people, when all these people may have needed, as a *very first step in their recovery*, is the chance to talk about how they feel, share their feelings in a non-judgmental setting, be shown how to go with the flow, be given non-invasive strategies to achieve self-awareness, and be given *time* to heal in a non-medicated way.

My advocacy for much-needed change is rooted in the fundamental rights of every person. Anyone who requires medical care has not only a responsibility to themselves, but the *right to choose* their health and life outcomes *without their end goals being imposed* by a third person (e.g. a doctor). I've spent too long working in the health, and allied health and safety, fields not to see practitioners and specialists (across many professional fields and especially in the areas of mental health, including my own staff), encourage a 'rely on me' attitude by their patients or clients, rather than encouraging their patients/clients to be self-reliant.

When a person's control is eroded or taken away by others, they are being robbed of what is rightfully theirs. And when it comes to psychic injuries in particular, the very personal nature of the responses makes it even more of an imperative that you have control of the process of recovery and healing. No-one knows how you feel and think better than you. No-one will ever know, and therefore the decisions you make that affect your life, *are for you to make.*

Being accountable means you are owning your choices - owning your behaviours, your words, and also owning what you don't do. It's inappropriate for you, or anyone else, to blame post-traumatic stress symptoms for your bad behaviour. Your behaviour is *always* your choice. For instance, for a court to allow post-traumatic-stress symptoms to be used as an excuse for murder or assault, is not only contradictory to the nature of acute stress reactions or post-traumatic stress symptoms (none of which include being aggressive towards others) it's also not laying the accountability for actions *on the individual who acted out a personal choice*.

From my own experience, at NO time did I ever consciously plan or act to hurt someone else because of the emotional responses I was experiencing. Where I might have felt like lashing out during episodes of what I (then) saw as pre-menstrual syndrome, I never acted on my feelings of anger. Because so many of our negative actions are founded in emotional baggage and pain that we carry, and only 'few' people have an uncontrolled desire to hurt others, the more I hear of PTSD being blamed for someone's bad behaviour, or their doing grave harm to another person, the more I know how deficient our legal justice systems are. Emotional responses don't make you choose to hurt someone. That choice and attitude to hurt is entirely separate, in my opinion.

Accountability is founded in responsibility, but it doesn't mean that all the responsibility lies with you. Within the context of your recovery and healing, determining who has responsibility for what aspects is fundamental to being able to delineate lines of accountability (ownership). A rehabilitation program will give each of the stakeholders their 'swim lanes', i.e. areas of responsibility and accountability, but the overarching subject of the rehabilitation (the rehabilitee) is you! A rehabilitation program has to be about you and your outcomes, first and foremost, even if other parties (such as your employer) have their part to play and their own lane to swim in.

CHAPTER 5

Utilizing personal growth and improved self-awareness as a vehicle for recovery and healing

Let's imagine for a moment that there is no such thing as the term "post-traumatic stress". Let's do away with the DSM and medical dictionaries and look at purely what's happening to you - the types of emotional responses or related physical symptoms that could still be impacting your life months or years after an event has passed:

- persistent nightmares or other sleep disturbances;
- flashbacks (images of the past event that come to your consciousness without warning) or other intrusive thoughts;
- intense emotional responses including prolonged feelings of fear, anxiousness (e.g. when imagery or sounds remind you of the event), or numbness;
- not maintaining eye contact;
- overactivity (in order to suppress your feelings or thoughts);
- being wary of your surroundings e.g. the people, the things happening/movements, the sounds;

- unrelenting desire to maintain control of everything;
- a change in your interpersonal skills leading to adverse effects on work, social, family or intimate relationships;
- severe loss of memory or concentration;
- substance abuse;
- episodes of or cyclic depression;
- social withdrawal.

It's not really relevant how many, or few, of these responses you are experiencing, it's more that the responses are (i) still there and (ii) impacting your life *in the present*. As well, your prolonged responses may also be impacting others in your family or inner sanctum and it is, unfortunately, a known fact that immediate family members can also be traumatized simply by watching what their loved one is going through after a traumatic event is over.

The traumatic event will likely have had deep reaching effects on your life and you may well have a sense of being very different than you were before the event. Well, in reality that is true – the event has changed you, both on the inside and the outside - and acknowledging and accepting this for what it is will help you to gain a deeper understanding of yourself and what it means to be human.

In Chapter 3 you may recall I raised the topic of our formative years and upbringing, and how these can influence our coping skills and overall makeup later in life. Where in this chapter the focus is going to be on two key things – understanding your prolonged emotional responses, and achieving personal growth and improved self-awareness - it's important to realize that your achieving these milestones is going to be directly influenced by your life pre-event, particularly the coping skills you learned during childhood.

Managing your response to or injury from a traumatic event is no different, in terms of your coping skills, than managing a crisis. Any crisis has the capacity to create stressors, usually extreme stressors, and management of those stressors requires a clear head, calmness, maintaining a sense of control and balance, and strong personal decision-making. However when management of the stressors is prolonged you will likely become quite fatigued, if not exhausted, at both a mental and emotional level. Based on my own experience post-trauma, and having experienced prolonged responses many years after some events, I do believe that when you get to that point of feeling emotionally or mentally exhausted, that's the point at which you can tip from 'acute trauma (crisis) management mode' into 'stressor management mode', and your "symptoms" can begin to become an everyday part of life.

Acknowledging and then understanding your emotional responses is a bit like checking your emotional health temperature. Recognizing within yourself that you are experiencing prolonged and stressor-related symptoms is the first step in your road to a healthier and happier living. Not judging yourself harshly is the second most important step. Beyond that, everything else is going to be governed by time, your level of self-motivation and desire for a positive self-fulfilling prophecy, and what support systems and people you can put in place to help you when you need it most.

When an event happens and even more so when you sustain an injury from the event, whether directly or indirectly, a number of things could be lost – time, control, a part of you, a life, a part of someone else, your surroundings, your home and other valued treasures, your family structure, your community, or even your safety. That loss, no matter how small or large, becomes a factor in how you are responding to the event and how long your response(s) will continue.

Grief is a normal process enabling you to come to terms with loss. You will grieve differently than other people; no two people grieve in exactly the same way as grief is completely relative to the depth of a loss. For instance, loss usually has a greater impact on people if it is unexpected, sudden or involves a child, and the initial response is usually one of total disbelief and shock.

Over the weeks and months that follow a loss you may experience waves of sadness, heartache and mental images of the person, and also suffer insomnia, loss of appetite, loss of interest and poor concentration. These are all normal responses.

From my own experience I know that enduring a major loss in my early adult years and having to then grieve that loss, was harder for me at an emotional level than dealing with other aspects of the traumatic event. In relation to that particular event, which occurred when I was 24, circumstances at the time were complicated by my not having an adequate support system and sufficient dialogue with key decision-makers pre-event and therefore, when the event occurred (which I initiated and ultimately had to hold only myself fully accountable for) my responses to that event were more intense than I could ever have imagined, and profoundly negative in their repercussions on my emotional and physical health.

Because we know that most traumatic events usually involve losing control of how our life is tracking, that is also going to be a large contributor to many of the other responses you might feel months or years afterwards. When we think we've lost control or, because of the event we actually do momentarily lose control over how life is going, the feelings of loss of control can turn to frustration, and frustration to anger and resentment. From there, the corrosive nature of anger (which is a negative energy in the body anyway[xlvii]) can lead to a range of physical symptoms. In a worst case scenario that anger can actually cause harm to the body at a cellular level.

Recognizing and *accepting* that all your responses are valid, true and real, even though the event may have long passed, is essential to your healing from that event. When you deny how you feel or don't pay enough attention to the signs and symptoms your body is giving you, then the responses will simply stick around. Denying your feelings won't make those feelings go away.

Another important point is that everything is relative. Nothing about a traumatic event, and how it impacts you emotionally, should be viewed in isolation. All the event factors are interlinked and therefore making sense of all of those factors is an important step in your recovery. Making sense of why the event happened (what went wrong to make it happen), how the event has changed you and why, all contribute to understanding your responses.

This is where root cause analysis comes in. When you understand the event and its root causes, even to the most basic of levels, this will automatically *inform your understanding* of your own responses, and in one of two ways. In simplistic terms, root cause analysis of an event is done to ensure that the event doesn't happen again. *If the event is something you contributed to or was in your control,* then your own analysis of it is an important part of learning lessons from your mistakes. *If the event wasn't in your control,* then when someone else identifies the root causes of it this will help provide context to why you feel the way you do.

Root causes are the underlying (fundamental) and reasonably identifiable reasons (i.e. causes) for an occurrence of 'something'.

In the context of understanding your prolonged emotional responses to an event long past, perhaps starting with my definition (of root cause analysis in this context) will help you understand why the process can help you:

> "a structured method used to determine and understand the causes of prolonged, adverse emotional responses to an unplanned event, with the aim of preventing continuation of the responses and a return to normal emotional functioning."

The analysis step can't take place without first identifying the root causes (of your emotional responses and apparent dysfunction) in the context of:

- the event;
- your holistic health (pre and post-event);
- your lifestyle (pre and post-event);
- your familial construct (pre and post-event); and
- your environment (pre and post-event).

Once you know the event's root causes (even at a basic level as I explained before), your goal should always be to investigate specific underlying causes for each of your emotional responses, one by one, remembering that some responses will be interlinked with others.

The majority of time spent doing root cause analysis is in gathering facts and filtering whether the facts are actual *causal factors that influence or direct an outcome, and can be fixed*, or just extraneous information that has no effectual reason associated with it. The whole idea of root cause analysis is to learn what caused your feelings to become so prolonged, and to remove those causal factors *with care* and without further delay. To do this effectively you must be prepared for some self-exploration and to accept that you may have made some mistakes, or misjudged something, and be willing to learn from your mistakes.

Self-acceptance of yourself in the now (the "I'm OK the way I am" philosophy) is a start. If you aren't seeing your own emotional responses as they currently are, as valid and true, then you've already put yourself in the victim/back seat not the driver's seat.

When you've gotten to the point of months or years past an event it almost becomes irrelevant *when* the event actually occurred. The event is way in your past and you've got to focus on how you feel *now*, acknowledging and accepting your responses for what they are. Why? Because:

- there's a whole lot of stuff that's gone on in your life since the event – some of it will possibly have been made worse because of your responses, some of it will be better, and some of the things that have gone on will be a direct result of your own responses;

- you are different now to before you were traumatized – life has moved on, even if you may not have moved as quickly with it – and yesterday, last week, last month and that event are already in your past. You can't change the past, only learn from it;

- at a physiological level you are different – you are older, and cellular changes have occurred whether you like it or not;

- you are already more experienced! By virtue of living another day, you've gained more experience. Without experience there's no way you could ever learn and improve on your coping skills, and develop resilience.

Often times when looking at causal factors the most visible, or obvious, things are focused on the most. For instance, a sleep disturbance like insomnia might be seen to be caused by living in a noise street, when in fact *one of the real causal factors* might be having too much information in your head (for the mind to successfully process the information subconsciously while you sleep) therefore keeping you awake. Depressive states might be seen to be caused by the loss of someone you loved, and missing them, when in fact *one of the real causal factors* might be that who've lost a sense of purpose in your life.

The causal factors that you need to look for are all those factors (some below the surface) that, once removed or resolved at an emotional level, will actually *eliminate or significantly reduce the severity* of negative feelings and responses. You might think that there's only one root cause for everything, but in the emotional realm I could almost guarantee that that is not true. The interlinkages of our emotional responses to things is one reason, and the importance of our emotions is another. When only one causal factor is identified and analyzed, then the ways to remedy the situation will be limited to one course of action. When all of the possible causal factors are identified for *each* of the individual responses, and then mapped to see if (and if so, how) they contribute to or are interdependent of each other, then the results will give you a loud and clear understanding of yourself, how you feel and how your body responds to those feelings.

Further, each causal factor you identify might have its own causal factors, so drilling down layer by layer is critical in understanding what caused what, or if what appears to be the root causal factor is actually just a symptom of another deeper causal factor.

In my first book *No Boxing Allowed*[xlviii] I talk at length about this process and how, in seeking to understand yourself and how you respond to things and why, this is the most powerful and courageous tool you can ever gift to yourself. Self-exploration and personal growth takes courage, commitment, unwavering determination to find answers, and a willingness to face the truths you uncover.

I give some simple examples in *No Boxing Allowed* about how to explore why we feel certain ways at certain times and what the underlying reasons are for how we feel and therefore what we do.

One relevant example is about a person who has to deliver some really bad news to someone else. The sequencing of questions allows you to explore why you feel a certain way, and to then drill down further and further until you get to the real root of the issue:

"*Scenario Two:* You have to deliver some bad news to someone and feel awful for being the messenger. You know they are very distressed as a result of the news.

Why are you feeling bad about delivering the message?
"Because I would rather someone else do it."

Why would someone else doing it make it any easier on the person receiving the news?
"It wouldn't, it would just get me off the hook."

Why do you want to be off the hook?
"Because I don't like delivering bad news, only good news."

Why is that?

"I don't know; maybe it's because when people have delivered bad news to me they seemed not to care how I felt."[xlix]

****

Strong roots usually run very deep and, just like a tree, roots can be a combination of superficial, surface (quick gratification) roots, or deep tap roots that travel to the core to gain access to long-term sustenance. Those nutrients can become polluted though, in which case the roots will deliver something that is damaging not only to the tree's actual integrity, but to how it functions and appears. If you think of your emotional responses as the leaves of a tree, flowing freely and easily, and how the leaves are fed by nutrients that originate from what the roots are gathering in from both the surface and also beneath the ground, you can see how a malfunction in the leaves is not likely to be the result of *just one* causal factor.

Once the causal factor fact-gathering is complete and then collated, and any interdependencies marked, you can then display the findings in a way that makes most sense to you e.g. a decision flowchart, a cause and effect table, a circuit diagram, or a route map, and so on. At that point you will have something quite tangible to work from.

Remember, whilst ever you are simply sitting, enduring your responses, not doing any reflective learning and self-exploration, then you're not choosing to sit in the driver's seat. The pain signal that I spoke about before, the body's last ditch hope to get through to you that something's still not quite right, is going to be right there in your face. It may come in the form of emotional pain (even heart pain), feeling sad all the time, recurring nightmares, unrelenting headaches, or even a noticeable physical pain whenever you're feeling really fearful. Whatever that pain signal is – be it mental, emotional or physical – don't ignore it! Recognize it, accept it and work to understand where it comes from. Take control of your outcomes by first taking that step towards self-awareness.

Once you have achieved a good understanding of your responses and their causal factors, deciding what to do next and in what order is the next major step. In all that I have experienced I know, without doubt, that your inner voice will tell you what should happen first, and then what next, in what sequence. You must be prepared to rely on your own intuitive gifts when making these decisions, as no-one knows you better than you. Some people might say they know you better than you, but (frankly) that's just BS. You're living in your skin and you're the one who's survived throughout life. You are your own 'expert'. Never forget that!

Living an authentic life is about knowing, and owning, who you are. Other people don't have to like you, but so long as you are true to who you really are, live authentically (not falsely), stay honest about yourself and know that you're not perfect, then you can freely like and love yourself, and not have to get permission from other people!

If you are doubtful about choosing a way forward with your recovery and healing at any time, then just pause a while. Don't procrastinate, just pause. There is a difference. One is indecision-based, the other is discernment-based.

Every decision you make about recovering and healing post-trauma should be discernment-based. Being discerning in your decisions and choices means being enlightened, informed and refined. Wait for more information to come to the surface, go back and reassess causal factors, listen to your body and the emotional responses you are feeling and assess whether something might be different now. If so, think about what's changed. TRUST yourself. Every decision that you make, at any point in time, will be the right decision *at that point in time*. Stop second-guessing yourself as that will only lead to indecision and the cycle will continue.

Don't opt for a second-best option when your health is the single most important thing in your life. Without good health you really have nothing. Every aspect of your quality of life is founded in your health. When your health is poor, your life will follow suit.

If poor health stops you from doing things, then you're missing out, aren't you? So, if you have to choose between poor and good health then always choose good health support options.

****

I'm going to finish this chapter with a story that highlights how important emotions and memories are.

You may not like some of your emotions and memories at the moment however when you see both of them as essential to living a complete life, you will learn to appreciate the gift that they are giving you. Using the gift of time, and opportunities that time creates, then a positive path forward can be locked on your 'radar screen of possibilities'. When the positive light stays on, the way is always clear. If you choose to switch that light off, then you (and only you) are responsible and accountable for finding the 'on' switch again.

Phineas Gage, 1823-1860, is history's most well-known brain injury survivor and a neuroscience miracle. A 1995 article in The Canberra Times[l] explains how the catastrophic head injuries sustained by Phineas in an industrial accident in 1848 (at age 25), including damage to his ventromedial prefrontal cortices, initially seemed not to affect him. Within a few minutes of the 13 pound metal bar blasting through his cheek and out through the top of his head, Phineas was walking and talking again. The article says "His memory, language, knowledge and attention span were all intact. Gradually, however, his friends began to notice that the Phineas Gage who emerged from the accident was a wholly different creature to the Phineas Gage they had known."

"Gage had been a shrewd and resourceful man, whose decisions could seldom be faulted. He emerged capricious, obstinate, rude and incapable of making sensible plans for his future. He was sacked from his job and fell in with bad company."

According to a Smithsonian website article [li] Gage's attending physician for the few months after the accident, John Martyn Harlow, "Gage's friends found him "no longer Gage"" and the balance between his "intellectual faculties and animal propensities" seemed gone. Harlow is said to have further written that Gage could not stick to plans, uttered "the grossest profanity" and showed "little deference for his fellows." After Gage's company not taking him back, Gage went to work at a stable in New Hampshire, drove coaches in Chile and eventually joined relatives in San Francisco, where he died in 1960, aged 36, after a series of seizures.

The Canberra Times' article explains "Others, who have lost the same region of the brain through less dramatic means – such as tumours or strokes – can display even more striking contradictions. While they may remain polite, alert, witty and coherent, they suffer from two pronounced deficiencies: a lack of feelings or emotions and a complete inability to make good or timely decisions. They can spend hours trying to decide which of two doors they should enter. Whatever mistake they make, they seem never to be able to learn from them."

It goes further to explain "Antonio Damasio, a professor of neurobiology, (says) that the two capacities – reason and emotion – are inextricably entwined. There are so many options inherent in every decision that we need some means of short-circuiting them if we're to do anything but sit in stupefied irresolution. Emotion and feeling are the tools we use. Experience – either rooted in childhood or more recent – associates the available options with either positive or negative emotions. At least in the early stages of making a decision, we are drawn towards one possibility as more attractive than its rivals through warmth of feeling.

The ventromedial prefrontal cortex is one of the places in the brain in which reason and emotion could be said to intersect. The poor souls who have lost theirs are left without any emotional involvement in decision-making, and are lumbered with working everything out by means of what Descartes would have described as reason: the isolated workings of a coldly calculating brain. They might take an age to make what we would recognise as an obvious choice or they might never get there at all, as they become enmeshed in the labyrinth of their analysis. They seem to have lost the ability to learn from past mistakes.

The brain, it appears, is constantly asking the body what it thinks. By reading the responses of our hearts, lungs, muscles and guts to a particular situation, it gets a rough idea of whether we like it nor not. Having eliminated most of the options in this way, it can then finish off the decision by what we know as logical means.

The brain's association with the body should not be altogether surprising. In our evolutionary past, decisions (such as whether to fight or flee) were made not by means of cost-benefit analysis, but through the biological response to stimuli. Reason, coming later, built on these foundations. Yet the presumed separation of mind and substance still dominate our assessment of ourselves.

What Damasio seems to have demonstrated is that human beings are irreducible. Our minds – or selves and souls – inhabit not an isolated part of us, but emerge from the interaction of brain, body and experience."

The Canberra Times article then goes on to explore how computers will never be able to think like humans. Where those in the computer industry claim that one day humans shall "soon create thinking computers which will have no emotions "only wisdom and knowledge"...If Damasio is right, wisdom is inextricable from emotion" (and) "Most importantly, Damasio's work appears to demonstrate that when humans try to behave as Daleks they are reducing, not extending, their capabilities.....We must heed those whose reason seems to be mediated by compassion and sympathy, rather than hatred and fear. Our hearts should tell us that any other choice would be illogical."

CHAPTER 6

Resilience for Life

resilience	In medicine, nursing and allied health fields:
	L, *resilere,* to spring back
	the ability of a body to return to its original form after being stretched or compressed.[lii]
	In the context of emotional resilience:
	* (MW) an ability to recover from and adjust easily to misfortune or change.
	Other generic definitions:
	* (O) the capacity to recover quickly from difficulties; toughness.
	* (MW) the ability to become strong, healthy and successful again after something bad happens.
	* (C) able to quickly return to a previous good condition.

For nearly 40 years, through many house moves and a few refrigerators, I have kept taped to my home refrigerator in Australia a quote by Wilfred A Peterson. I have absolutely no recollection of where I got it, whether it was in a magazine or a newspaper, but the words are presented nicely in a decorative box. The reason I keep it taped to the refrigerator is to teach others. The quote rings as true to my life now as it did back in the early 80's when I first found it. In 1983 my Australian son was born and being a good and effective parent was something I was determined to be, despite experiencing poor parenting within my own family construct as a child. The quote from Peterson also quotes John Donne:

"The Art of Parenthood

 "Of all the commentaries on the Scriptures", wrote John Donne, "good examples are best".

Our children are watching us live, and what we are shouts louder than anything we can say.

When we encircle them with love they will be loving.

When we are thankful for life's blessing they will be thankful.

When we express friendliness they will be friendly.

When we speak words of praise they will praise others.

When we set an example of honesty our children will be honest.

When we practice tolerance they will be tolerant.

When we confront misfortune with a gallant spirit they will learn to live bravely.

When our lives affirm faith in the enduring values of life they will rise above doubt and scepticism.

We can't stand there pointing our finger to the heights we want our children to scale.

We must start climbing and they will follow."

Its messages are simple yet so powerful, and good examples *are* always best. I was fortunate to have maternal grandparents who, by default, taught me how parenting should be, and they lived this quote in every way. They were my most influential roles models during my childhood and, despite the many traumas that I endured out of their sights, their positive attitude and underlying values were what (I know) helped nurture my resilience.

One of the fundamental things about developing resilience is that you have to experience things first! Without experiences to expand our minds, and hone our coping skills, we might just as well be content to be a slug in the garden. Emotional resilience is founded in living a healthy, balanced life; learning things; applying those learnings; learning from our mistakes; and having strong, bonding relationships with others that can withstand obstacles and tests that we face in life.

In that sense then, the very first challenging experience you had in your life as a baby was the beginning of your journey in building your resilience. Throughout your childhood no doubt you experienced many more things, each of these adding to your repertoire of coping skills and acting to mature you at an emotional level. With motivation to do better next time, you would have honed your coping skills, building emotional and mental strength as you grew.

I'm sure you would have observed quite a few people in your life whom you felt didn't 'cope very well'. The kind of folks you would likely think of as 'not being very resilient'. Well, those folks are still on their journey (like you are) so it's best not to judge them too harshly. Where some people never seem to grow up, or grow any gumption to pick themselves up after falling, or have the courage to take control of their outcomes, or sit around feeling sorry for themselves, if nothing else you must realize one thing. *YOU can't change them. They have to want to change, strengthen and improve themselves.*

As I've said earlier, you are in control of the choices that you make as opportunities present themselves. You are the one who can choose to be the driver of your life, or sit back and be a passenger. I've known so many passengers in my life if I wrote a book about each of them (and averaged 2 months per book) I'd be writing for at least the next 100 hundred years. SO many people who had such huge potential but wasted their lives wallowing in self-pity and playing the victim card. So many people!

No matter *what* life dishes out, you have an opportunity to make something good come of every experience and build more emotional strength at the same time. No matter what. No exceptions. No excuses.

In this chapter, I'm focused on giving you both reassurance and tips. How you run with those tips, or measure your achievements to date, is up to you. Regardless of whether life is a struggle for you at the moment, or whether you may have reached a cross-roads and aren't quite sure what road to take next, never underestimate just how capable you are of making a decision, and living with the consequences of that decision (be they good or bad). You have the wherewithal to make positive change in your life, and as you make those changes you will be building your resilience for the future. The power is with you!

****

Generally speaking, highly resilient people are aware of situations and how these situations impact them at a personal level, they understand that they will have an emotional response to some situations more deeply than other situations, they know the strategies to get themselves back into life again afterwards, and they also understand the behaviour and responses of others (to those situations), a lot better than those people who aren't so resilient.

As you build resilience your coping skills may vary from time to time when confronting each situation. This may be due to the situation being more severe or life-changing than a previous situation, and you're not quite sure what to do and not do, or it may just be that you aren't feeling as up to handling things at that time in your life. Maybe something in how you feel or something about your life may not give you that extra bit of support you need to knuckle down and face the issues. Maybe there are too many situations all coming at once. Only you will have true context, so it would be wise to *be kind to yourself* while you work it all out.

While people vary widely in how they cope with crisis situations, there are some fundamental, key characteristics to building resilience and living a life with confidence in your own abilities. Building on your coping skills each time, focusing on learning lessons from the past while looking and walking forward to the future, are all pivotal in helping you to tackle things with innovation and flexibility, and grow stronger in managing your emotional responses. The above pure definitions are a good starting point for understanding what resilience is and the following tips will assist you to achieve a healthy level of resilience, however *enduring emotional resilience (i.e. resilience for life)* should be your ultimate goal.

Strong coping skills and high levels of resilience are characterized by:

* **maintaining awareness of and relativity to surroundings** – within the context of the situation and your level of control over some or all aspects, maintaining awareness of yourself (and how you are feeling) within the environment created by the situation, coupled with taking as much control as possible of how the situation pans out, will assist in empowering you to move forward, assess risks in a discerning manner and make sound, informed decisions.

When you have zero control of a situation, then maintaining awareness of how you are responding to the situation and the changes it brings, will help you to rationalize the event after it has passed.

Once the situation subsides (or the event passes) re-group mentally and emotionally and start visualizing yourself in the *now*, not in the past.

* **being open, adaptable and flexible** – understanding that life is full of challenges, setbacks, decisions and changes, a number of which are not going to be in your control, is essential to:

- minimizing internal stressors,
- staying relatively relaxed and calm during decision-making,
- maintaining mental clarity,
- being emotionally intelligent about what's happening and other people's responses,
- going-with-the-flow, rather than fighting, resisting or losing your cool, and
- thriving after the situation has passed.

In a danger situation people often become tunnel-vision and mentally and emotionally rigid. Whilst this is a normal survival response in some situations, it can lead to you patterning the same response behaviour at other times which might not warrant such a fixated view.

When you are being overly tunnelled in your view of things, you'll miss facts that could potentially be very critical to your recovery and healing, and ability to thrive, afterwards.

* **being self-motivating, self-reliant and resourceful** – "Don't look to others to motivate you. Others can inspire you, but the strongest and most sustainable motivation comes from within."[liii]

As we explored earlier, self-reliance is not about relying solely on yourself at all times but rather about helping yourself first rather than always looking to others for support (especially with small, easy things). If you can achieve something on your own that's a more empowering posture to adopt, than always reaching out for help and leaning on others.

Resilience is honed by gradually increasing the level of challenges faced and conquering them using ingenuity and resourcefulness.

* **a capacity and willingness to make a decision and stick with it** – indecisiveness and lack of tenacity have the capacity to become your worst Archilles' heel, if you let them. Life isn't a test, but life *is* a series of experiences that

come as a direct result of either (i) choices that we make or (ii) unexpected events that occur without a conscious choice being made by us to be involved.

When you make a wilful choice that turns out to be not-so-good, hopefully you'll learn from your mistake. If the choice gives you a good result, then kudos to you for being that little bit more discerning to begin with.

When an unplanned traumatic event creates an experience that you'd rather not have endured, then obviously the choice factor is not something you could necessarily have controlled. Your commitment to being decisive and tenacious is going to be influenced by how much that event impacted you, either directly or indirectly.

* **applying a solution and outcome-oriented approach** - don't shy away from solving small, seemingly innocuous dilemmas, as 'practice makes perfect' and when a large, daunting challenge comes along you'll be better prepared and more able to sustain the mental and emotional focus necessary to tackle it head on.

Simply waiting for a challenge to go away on its own only prolongs the situation and the inevitability of having to make a decision.

Coming up with solutions, rather than focusing on what's going wrong, will help you to both recover quicker and be empowered to take full control of your life again, when the time is right. In the face of a challenge, one strategy could be to make a quick list of potential ways to solve the situation and then work each potential solution through to the end outcome, using a scenario building approach. Focus on good outcome scenarios (positive self-fulfilling prophecies), rather than bad.

* **maintaining healthy relationships with significant others** – when your inner sanctum is working constructively and cooperatively together, decision-making is less stressful and more discerning, and compromises can be reached without delay.

In life, aside from your health the rest of life is all about 'relationships'. A good barometer reading of the health of your most important and meaningful relationships will show clearly that emotional pressures are minimal and cooperation is high; active listening is deployed by all; and compassion and respect (founded on trust, which is founded on truth[liv]) go hand-in-hand with each other.

* **maintaining strong social connections** – whenever you're are dealing with situations or having to make important decisions, it's vital to have the right people around who could offer support if needed. Likewise have solid friends to whom you can simply offload (vent) a little – without dumping – is important to achieve balance in your life. When life is sitting square on your shoulders and the weight gets too much to bare at times, there's absolutely nothing wrong with sharing.

Talking through strategies and options with your support network is also a healthy way to make sure your action plan is balanced and discerning. Sometimes third and fourth opinions are good, just like getting a quote for maintenance of your home, collecting a range of views from people you trust is usually far healthier than going it entirely alone.

Having a friendly, caring network of supporters is particularly helpful when a major crisis presents, as that is the time when you are likely to need confidantes the most. In times of crisis they are more likely to give you positive, constructive advice and support, than add to your pressures.

* **being able to ask for help when needed** – there's nothing whishy-washy or wrong with asking for help. The strongest and most resilient people know that asking for help, when they really need it, is actually empowering to themselves *and others.*

Being self-motivating, self-reliant and resourceful is essential to growing your level of resilience however there may well be times when things just get too tough, rough or daunting. It's perfectly fine to say "enough" and reach out for help from professionals with particular training and knowledge in the issues that you are facing.

Attending useful seminars, workgroups, relaxation and meditation groups; being involved in legitimate on-line support groups; or undertaking some counselling, remedial therapies like massage or reflexology, or more targeted therapies (like hypnotherapy and cognitive behavioural therapy); can be both beneficial and liberating. The mere act of asking for help is a positive step – you are being proactive, staying in control and focusing on the future (not the past).

* **identifying as a survivor, not a victim** – in any situation that pushes you beyond your current coping skills or challenges you in a way that makes you re-evaluate life to some extent or another, it is essential to view yourself as a survivor, rather than a victim of circumstance. While a situation may be out of your control to change, looking forward whilst learning from what happened, will give you a positive motivation and place you more readily in the driver's seat where the future is yours to make choices about.

Giving control away to others may be necessary to bring about healing from a physical injury, however emotional injuries heal better when the injured is the one who is given and readily accepts control of life going forward.

* **a positive mindset** – staying positive during dark periods in life can be difficult, and at times seemingly impossible, but maintaining a sense of hope is fundamental to resiliency. Being positive doesn't mean ignoring bad things that go on, rather it means switching your focus away from the negative as soon as possible, and not staying wallowing in negative thoughts.

Negativity is a dark, energy-sapping place to be. Positivity equates to lightness, freedom and self-motivating energy. Staying optimistic about possibilities, and looking for the positive in opportunities and changes, once again keeps you focused on the future and walking forward.

99

A positive mindset will reinforce that change is a constant thing in life, that as one door might close another will open and time will always deliver more opportunities in due course, and that setbacks are transient. "Change is always an opportunity, never a threat."[lv]

* **holding faith in your own abilities** – I'm not talking about religious faith here; I'm talking about self-belief. When you believe in yourself, nothing will keep you down.

Granted sometimes you could feel like you've been hit by a freight train, however maintaining confidence that you have the intestinal fortitude and wherewithal to pick yourself up, dust yourself off, and have another go, will empower you like nothing else.

Self-esteem plays a huge role in your capacity to cope with life's stressors and when you've survived a traumatic event the first thing you need to acknowledge is that *you survived it*! That survival, alone, means you have achieved a positive outcome, and reminding yourself through self-affirmations and writing down your self-fulfilling prophecy, will bolster your strengths and support your accomplishments.

Having faith means really trusting yourself and believing that your inherent/innate (inborn, natural, permanent) abilities and characteristics are all that you need *at this point in time*. When you face adversity with faith in yourself, that mindset will automatically result in a greater level of resilience each time.

* **seeing setback as an opportunity to learn** – in *No Boxing Allowed* I introduced "there are no failures in life, only opportunities from which to learn and grow."[lvi] In reality a failure generally means a breakdown in how something was *meant to happen*. A setback is not that 'something' was meant to happen *and didn't*, it means an obstacle or a situation has altered the planned path of the 'something' (i.e. how it was tracking).

We can have all the plans in the world in life, but planning for all potential deviations from our plan, and having contingencies for all those potential deviations is nigh on impossible. Life for most people is full of surprises – some good, some bad. However 'rolling with the punches' of life and seeing each setback as an opportunity to re-evaluate the plan, and choose a new path, is a much more productive and positive way to view situations. Particularly when the setbacks are completely out of your control to influence or change.

* **maintaining a purpose in life** – whether you realize it or not, every human is placed on this earth for a reason. Seeing life as a gift, not to be squandered or taken for granted, is a not only a self-motivating approach but also an inspirational one.

Prior to a traumatic event, you may already have had a plan for your future and seen a purpose or direction to your life. If the event changed that, or your particular circumstances, so that you can't really fulfil that original purpose anymore, then look for a new path. Change direction a little.

When you know yourself really well - i.e. your current strengths, limitations and deficiencies – and you can envision the changes to make that can then allow you to build a new vision then you will automatically have given yourself a purpose. Whether you then choose to turn your talents and skills to help others, or set new dreams to accomplish for yourself, it doesn't really matter so long as the outcome requires you to live a directed, meaningful and outcome-oriented life.

* **a nurturing and self-loving posture** – destructive and self-harming behaviours can become common place after a traumatic event and it's critical that you keep an eye on this aspect very closely. If you know that you have these tendencies then seeking support from others (whether friends, family or suitable medical professionals) must be on your daily radar of self-awareness, until the feelings resolve and disappear.

When you give love to yourself and look after yourself holistically you are not only building the resilience bank account with healthy deposits, you're also subliminally programming your subconscious mind that *you are important and you deserve looking after*. Nurturing yourself isn't about pampering or giving yourself extras, and it's not about mothering yourself. It's about caring for, cherishing and protecting yourself. When you feel super tired, unmotivated, overwhelmed or overly emotional, it's very easy to stop eating, ignore exercise and not get enough sleep. When stressors are present it's very easy to neglect your own needs and put others first.

Focusing on programming your mind to always see nurturing yourself as essential, not optional, and taking time to do things that nurture your soul, will mean that when the next situation or crisis comes along you will be in the strongest and healthiest position to help yourself get through it.

* **being able to restore a sense of control without delay** – when a traumatic event occurs a highly resilient person will recognize very quickly that they've momentarily lost control but they won't hit the P button (i.e. the panic button). They will carefully, perhaps cautiously, and with discernment identify all the facts, determine strategies to improve on the situation and determine a way forward, without delay.

Where someone is building their resilience level, if they view a crisis situation as a permanent loss of control or are not able to see a way forward, this knock-on effect will only perpetuate negative thoughts and a negative outcome.

Any traumatic event will involve certain people or entities taking responsibility and being held accountable. What you're ultimately accountable for is achieving 'as best a future as possible under the prevailing circumstances' and remaining empowered to make your *own choices* to support that new future.

Resilience for Life is demonstrated in the capacity to get up stronger each time after being repeatedly knocked down; rise above the worst adversities and still stay smiling and confident; remain compassionate and forgiving in the wake of your worst enemies or adversaries' actions; and remain positive and self-affirming regardless of bad things that might be said about or to you.

The simple choices of:

- maintaining the goal of inner peace, making that your mindful choice every day; and
- writing down your prophecy and as many positive affirmations as you need – i.e. good and motivating messages about yourself - and putting these in view so that you can reflect on them from time to time,

will help create your self-fulfilling prophecy! The symptoms associated with Post-Traumatic Stress may be present in your life right now, but that is not to say that they always will be.

"Your destiny is yours to choose, not another's to dictate. Choose the destiny that resonates well for you. Find calmness and strength within, and .... think creative, inspirational and empowering thoughts."[lvii] And above all else, from this moment on, "don't put emotional energy into something that hasn't happened yet".[lviii]

CHAPTER 6

A Personal Reflection: a brief history of my own experiences with trauma

I am very pleased to be in a position to present my experiences in this book, reflected as examples through the previous chapters and also summarized here. To a certain extent this book echoes my first three books, so I do hope that this last chapter gives you some context to why I've quoted my "inspirational" first book, *No Boxing Allowed*, so often.

My fourth book *Feronia – The Little Girl Who Learned To Fly Free*, a children's book on thriving after trauma, is complementary to this one but also stands alone in that its target audience is 7-15 year olds. Where the two books discuss some different things, and at different levels of understanding, both are similar in reflecting the possibilities and challenges that traumatized people face.

My history with trauma dates back to my childhood, however despite the extraordinary number of traumatic events in my life, I can stand with hand on heart and know that I am fully healed from the residual impacts of those events. That 18-month period of intense healing work, 15+ years ago, was a turning point for me – I found even more courage at a time when I thought my courage had run out and my options were invisible.

I have never been a member of the military, or served as an employee in what I would call 'front-line' war-like scenarios. However, I have experienced many different kinds of traumatic and extreme risk events. Collectively, the events impacted me through all four dimensions – mentally, emotionally, physically, and spiritually - and therefore being able to view my post-trauma recovery and healing using a 'resilience lens' was absolutely essential to my survival, and quality of life afterwards.

Despite 2001-2 being a positive turning point, from 2002 wasn't easy by any stretch of the imagination. My son and I were both impacted by my leaving my marriage, the divorce in 2002 had a significant impact on him, and then the horrific plane crash which claimed his half-brother (Derek) in December 2005 devastated everyone. The immediate days and weeks following the crash were most difficult for me because I was grappling with not only my son's loss of his last surviving sibling, and dearly wanting to take his pain away, I was still coming to terms with the horror of the event myself.

Within weeks I reached out to a clinical psychologist to help me develop strategies to help my son, whilst still grieving myself. During the two 45 minute sessions in which she supported me, mainly by listening, I talked about a range of things and she questioned me about my past to get context to my high level of concern for my son. We also talked about the other siblings my son had lost.

The clinical psychologist summarized her view of me as 'incredibly resilient', and it would appear those foundational skills were first learned during my early childhood years. My coping skills and resilience grew over time as a direct result of both the events I survived and being put into positions of authority and responsibility at a very, young age. I could now appreciate that who I am today is testament to my ability to rise above adversity each and every time, find a positive in every situation, apply my lessons with courage and tenacity, and learn from my mistakes and those of others.

My life has been one where lessons came hard and there were usually significant risks and setbacks to face in applying the learning from those lessons. In many respects I am harder on myself than anyone else could ever dream to be and I don't cut myself near as much slack as I did when I was younger. I do hold a higher expectation of myself than for others, which is in part inspired by a deep spiritual awareness but also driven by a commitment to be there, where humanly possible, for others whom I know need me the most.

That is partly why I have dug up my past, to write this and my other books which I know can help others. But also, I've never seen, heard or read about any other books, other than this one, that's written by someone *who's actually had post-traumatic stress symptoms lasting a seriously long time, and fully healed from them.*

It is therefore without pride or prejudice that I share my experiences.

I've grouped them into two main types and trust that my interpretations help you to understand how I built on my resiliency after each situation had passed.

The two groups are:

(i)   those events that I recognized had a deep impact on me, either in the form of short or prolonged emotional responses, or resulted in some serious life lessons and changes; and

(ii)   those that were traumatic (by virtue of their scale) or very impactful for a period, but didn't result in any emotional *injury* to me as such. These events *include* where I was either 'available/on standby' (e.g. as a first aider) or summoned 'ad hoc' to come and assist the injured after a traumatic event had occurred.

****

(i)   My childhood began with my parents being separated, so the absence of a father figure was (for the observer) a potential set-back for me in not having a balanced upbringing in the immediate family dynamic. My birth was not something that either parent had planned for and, in that regard, I was already placed in the 'too hard basket' by the time I was born. That scenario introduced significant risks to my wellbeing, as you could imagine, and made navigation of the family dynamic very challenging and filled with emotional outbursts by the adults involved. As much as my grandparents provided an example of male-female balance when I was in their presence and care, they were not the sole guardians of my welfare. A range of pressures existed for my mother which unfortunately, as an unwanted child from the beginning, meant I bore the brunt of most of her deficiencies, biases and hatred and, as exhibited many times in her life, serious lack of coping skills. The clinical psych' I spent those two sessions with asked me some pointed questions about my childhood early in the second session and then congratulated me on 'parenting my own parent' while I was still a child. Without perhaps intending to, she caused me to consciously acknowledge my high level of resilience. She also reinforced to me how my having coped with my mother (and what I thought were my mother's adult-level emotional responses, when in fact they were responses typical of an unrestrained and misguided child), enabled me to build strong skills during my formative years and also function well despite the pressures that had been placed on me so young.

My childhood was punctuated with what I would call normal family dynamics – spending time with relatives of the same age, family and extended family outings – however there was a high level of physical abuse, mostly during period between 1 and 15 years of age. The 'punishments' were administered to me for a range of reasons - something I was believed to have done, as a result of my questioning a person directly about their horrible behaviour or objecting to being badly treated, and in some cases for what I could only fathom as 'just because'. The physical abuse caused emotional injuries as well, as on most occasions the punishment was not justified and the severity of the physical abuse would nowadays be classified as reportable. It was always a struggle for me to equate the reality of what I knew had or hadn't happened, with the treatment I was receiving. Nothing ever added up and my emotional response to the events was usually to withdraw, go quiet and avoid the aggressors as much as possible. Some of the worst events involved mental abuse by several family members and also abandonment by my primary carer (mother) during times of real and justifiable need. My mother did not seek timely medical attention for me on a couple of occasions (inflamed appendix being one) and this led to two traumatizing things – my mother avoiding visiting me in hospital, and doctor's isolating me in a specific hospital ward for a lengthy period post-op to ensure best possible recovery.

There were also pivotal events from around age seven, involving one of her boyfriends and one of my own uncles, which resulted in my strong feeling of fear, bad nightmares, flashbacks, and perpetual avoidance of people and situations. In this day and age the actions of the boyfriend would be called second-degree sexual misconduct involving a minor, and, for the uncle, inappropriate behaviour (suggestions and approaches). At the time I managed the threats they presented in a number of key ways – avoiding any contact with them where possible and (especially) working hard to not be left alone with them in a room; talking my way out of the situation by being as nice as possible to prevent them reacting with anger; and telling my mother about the incidents, none of which she appeared to believe and certainly did nothing to change. My emotional responses to these events varied and some lasted many years, until about my later teens. At this time I became aware that the bad feelings had definitely settled down and I was feeling much stronger and happier. In the case of the nightmares and flashbacks, by my early teens they had disappeared and I do believe this healing can be attributed to my being more mobile and away from the home environment, with far less threat contact than previously when I was much younger.

In reflecting on this period in my life I know full well my mother had no capacity or willingness to rationalize others' or her own negative behaviour towards me and resolve the root causes. The focus was never on solutions, rather on punishing and perpetuating the symptoms of a dysfunctional and abusive family dynamic.

As a result of her lack of empathy and relationship management skills, and complete disbelief of the concerns I was raising, my calls for assistance and support went unheeded during my entire childhood. I feel sure that her intense desire for control over my life was as debilitating for her as it was for me.

The next traumatic event in my younger years was around 18-19 years of age during a time when I was holding senior responsibility and accountability professionally (i.e. was performing in a senior leadership role at age 19) and also still doing professional modelling work (TV ads, major client product promotions on-site, and photographic and runway modelling). An elderly man lived near my modelling agent's house and, for whatever reason, I had to attend that house one day. Unfortunately he was deceased and his body was inside the house. The vision of seeing the body and smelling the initial smells of decomposition were the two things that stayed with me for quite a few months. I was deeply impacted by the fact that he was alone in the house for so long after he died, and that emotional response was the hardest for me to work through. In terms of residual responses, the negative ones included disturbed sleep for a while and also a sense of helplessness (that I hadn't found him alive in time). On the positive side it did reinforce in me the need to keep communicating with important people so that they felt loved and cared about. My grandparents were my strongest 'parent' role models and I was very close to them. This event, whilst a bad outcome for the gentleman in question, allowed me time to refocus on my grandparents whom, by that stage, were seeing less of me given that I had grown up, was 'busy' with my own life, and no longer in school and having regular holidays with them.

At age 23, a couple of months prior to finding out I was going to be immigrating to the USA (sponsored by an American-Irish multinational company) I started dating a professional athlete (football player). He seemed to be a reasonable human being on the surface however, on attending at his home one evening I was met by not only him but two of his fellow housemates as well. Despite having been in a relationship with one man for the year prior to that time, a man whom I felt 100% safe with and who treated me the way a person deserves to be treated, as you could imagine my level of wariness of men was still fairly high and my distrust of men pretty consistent. Aside from the longer term partner, no man I'd ever known had ever been completely trustworthy or honourable, and I'd learned through my life that unsavoury men always used lies and manipulated situations to serve their purpose.

The sexual assault that ensued was not only a shock to me at every level, it destroyed the trust I had only started to build and, from an emotional impact level, put me squarely back on the batting plate, not even on life's 1st base.

The event knocked my self-esteem to pieces, my fear level increased again and I became hypersensitive to all male attention. This, unfortunately, is not something I found men could easily understand; that when a woman (or child) is manhandled inappropriately or sexually assaulted in a worst case scenario, the very thought of being with a man after that is not only nauseating, it can be downright terrifying.

Fortunately for me, the next man I had any close contact with after that event was in fact the man I'd been in a relationship with earlier, the "safe" man, so his very presence in my life again enabled a HUGE healing and trust building period for me. He was from the USA originally and had long since returned States-side. Having immigrated there myself just before my 24th birthday, at his invitation I had the opportunity to reacquaint and visit with him and his family/friends for a fortnight before I was to start my new job. The immigration/sponsoring aspects weren't altogether free of issues, given that a potential future boss showed all the signs of being a sexual predator, so the mere fact that I was now in the company of the "safe" man, a man I also still loved and held very positive memories of, that was my silver lining and my ray of hope for a "home run" outcome.

When in his company (particularly) I felt much protected, at a number of levels, and even when he was away for work for up to several weeks at a time, I still felt "safe" knowing that he was the one in my life. We lived together, I worked, he worked, and life was comfortable and nurturing for me until around the Christmas time of 1981. This was my first Christmas away from my home country and my beloved grandparents and that period spending time with his family, whilst enjoyable and fun on the one hand, was deeply distressing. I was physically separated from him at night, at a time when I needed to maintain a sense of closeness and bonding. He was the only person I felt I could truly trust to support my growing sense of wholeness and wellbeing.

I felt betrayed and controlled by this situation of separation, a very similar sentiment to how I had felt about my own mother and her controlling ways, and unfortunately this caused some of the old bad memories of my mother to resurface.

During that period States-side I also had a serious woman's health issue to deal with mid-January 1982 (in the middle of one of their coldest winters), which required emergency transportation to hospital one night and then follow up surgery. The surgery was meant to have left me sterile for up to 6 months BUT that didn't turn out to be the case. I fell pregnant within weeks of the surgery.

The pregnancy was an unplanned situation but one that made me very happy after I got the news, because most importantly I dearly loved that man and wanted to have his child, even though that had not been a plan we spoke of, and also our mutual friends whom I shared the news with were very happy too. They knew being a mom would be good for me and the child.

However, the next couple of months proved to be not quite so favourable and my elation and hopefulness ultimately turned in the other direction. The next weeks of medical consultations, talking with doctors, attempting to find a solution on my own were mentally and emotionally draining, physically intrusive, and spiritually eroding. Not only was there minimal discussion with or comment from him (largely given his shock of such major news and also him being offshore and unable to communicate in private ship-to-shore), I was also isolated from my grandparents (and had no way of quickly communicating with them and getting advice), had no desire to involve my controlling mother in the conversation, and I didn't feel that his family would support me either, given his negative sentiment on hearing the news.

I walked forward, hesitating at many times, in what I know was an emotional fog of confusion, fear, and helplessness, and had my pregnancy terminated under the worst possible emotional conditions. The termination procedure not only caused internal injury to me, which later produced complications for me in conceiving, carrying to term and having a scar-free uterus, it was my pivot point into the darkest of dark emotional tunnels and resulted in some post-traumatic stress symptoms being present over the next almost two decades.

I will say that my prolonged emotional responses were not 24/7 – some symptoms would subside for months and even years, while others surfaced, and they'd cycle like that over the years depending on the triggers of the past. Further, the emotional injury caused by the termination was certainly exacerbated by a number of other key factors and events:

- having to return to the home where I lived with him, minus my unborn child;
- not seeing him face-to-face until after the termination was over and him seeming to be regretful;
- a few months later splitting from him; then
- leaving the States to come back to Australia (and that was definitely not what I had seen coming when I immigrated);
- rushing into a new relationship on the rebound, that enabled me to fall pregnant and quickly replace the baby I had lost;
- subsequently marrying the father of my new child when I subconsciously knew that wasn't going to make things better for me and, of course, then living in what eventually became an unfulfilling and dysfunctional marriage, one which was also mentally and emotionally damaging; and lastly
- finding out that the scar my son was born with (a birthmark on his face) was malignant.

In my autobiography *The Peace Angel*, which was first published and launched in 2014 and has since won 17 awards, I talk at length about that long period of my life and the lessons I learned. It will serve no direct purpose to rehash all of that here, and so I will leave you with this one statement:

Ending the life of a child in utero is bad enough. Ending the life of a child that you wanted with all your heart, and a child made with a man whom you knew was the love of your life, is not just traumatic, it's soul destroying. The ensuing decades of torment, heartache, grief and sorrow were endured as a result of two life-changing losses at once – the baby, and him.

My healing from that long period of immense challenge came initially in 2001, when I decided to leave my marriage (more on that in (ii)), followed by some facilitated hypnotherapy. From 2003, after I gained qualifications in clinical hypnotherapy myself to understand the science of the mind and how the conscious mind syncs with memories, I followed on with self-hypnosis on a nightly basis for the first couple of years, then as-needed, until around 2006. My self-hypnosis helped me to reprogram my mind to reject prolonged negative thoughts which effectively means I can't, repeat can't, stay negative in my thinking even after the worst disaster, trauma or crisis situation. Giving myself the power to bounce back to the positive with greater speed than before, using my thought processing as the vehicle, was the only way I could see walking forward in life and having control over how other people's negative actions and words would impact me.

The result of my efforts are profoundly positive however the only downside is that sometimes people see me as being superficial in my feelings. This is a shame because I still feel things very deeply, am affected by some things at a profound level, but the sad feelings and any emotional baggage has no chance of sticking around. I have long realized this is my ultimate emotional survival 'gift' I gave to myself - reprogramming my mind to the positive, and permanently exfoliating all my life-long emotional baggage.

Of course, I still retain some memories of negative people and events as these memories are "essential" to my survival. The memories definitely help to prevent me from being exposed to people in my past who proved themselves to be a threat to my wellbeing. Some of those people have since died, some are still around somewhere, but regardless of where they are and what they're doing, they are now inconsequential to my existence and not part of my life. The memory of them is there but it's devoid of any 'emotional' connection (or pain).

(ii)   By the time I was 15 I believe I'd developed some pretty robust coping skills and this was demonstrated in the middle of the night one night, when a motorcyclist was involved in a crash with a car right outside my bedroom window. I remember going outside and comforting that cyclist, making him a cup of warm tea (to help with his shock), and the sight of his and other's injuries did not cause me to suffer any ill effects. My resilience, by that stage, had been reinforced by me staying positive and focusing on fun and lightness. I could have chosen to wallow and be unhappy but that was not my nature anyway, so I didn't. I always kept focused on a brighter future, no matter what it took to get there.

Prior to moving overseas in 1981 my beloved grandfather had become quite ill with Parkinson's Disease and, by the time I was 21 they were living in a smaller home nearby to their original seaside property. My grandmother was also sick with diabetes, though she seemed to be physically and emotionally more robust than he, and was coping quite well. When I returned from the USA, I helped myself by focusing on other things other than the baby and partner I'd lost. By this stage my grandfather was in a nursing home. He was not doing so well so I turned every negative situation I saw, into a positive action – taking him for outings, visiting him and talking together, visiting my grandmother and providing emotional support to her; being company to her in the retirement village where she lived alone. In those days my quiet sorrow at finding Pa isolated and ill, and Grandma alone, became a motivator for me to give back time to them, as they had given so readily to me as a child. If I could have lived with my grandmother then I would have, to help her in any way I could.

In late 1982 I met my future son's father and that meeting introduced some considerable stressors into my life – his angry estranged wife from whom he had already separated (for whatever strange reason I became the brunt of her hatred), his 12 year old daughter who was in remission again from fighting leukaemia, and his son Derek who was emotionally sensitive due to his parent's split and his sister's illness. I know I didn't take on their emotional baggage, at that time, firstly because I had enough of my own in those early months after my pregnancy ended and I wanted to be their 'carer' and comforter. That role empowered me to not get too lost in all the negatives that surrounded us.

I stayed strong even while things around us seemed to crash in every direction. When I fell pregnant around Christmas of 1982, the property settlement and divorce aspects were underway with his soon-to-be ex-wife and that introduced all sorts of new negatives into the family dynamic. This second (and last) pregnancy was fraught with 'morning sickness from hell' and threatened miscarriages on three separate occasions.

In early 1983 my stepdaughter (Toni) had undergone a bone marrow transplant after Derek had given his marrow, which meant that both of them were healing and needing emotional support. My fiancée and I, with me still struggling to stay pregnant with my new baby, supported the children via normal visitation rights and provided all the care we could. Financially things were atrocious, and that was an added strain. However, the worst event came in the May when we found out that Toni had come out of remission again and the doctors made clear there was nothing they could do. I went into early labor again (3-4 months premmy), arguments and strain became the norm in the household due to the health, financial and divorce aspects, and my mother's increasing pressure to be involved. Yet, through all that I know I didn't crumble, I kept the happy face in the family as my fiancée fell into gloom and frequent drinking episodes. I was flat out determined not to lose my unborn child even if it meant leaving and starting a new life on my own.

August 1982 was an upended month – my grandfather died in the second week and I gave birth to my son on the 20th (3 weeks early). I couldn't get to my grandfather's funeral which made me very sad, but I remember staying as focused and forward-looking as I could. My son was taken from me for many hours in the hospital and 'misplaced' - that was not a pleasant few hours to endure! Toni was becoming quite physically incapacitated by then, often in a wheel chair (until she permanently became wheelchair and bed bound in the September). Keeping the family environment buoyant and lively was my key aim. I didn't want my newborn facing more pressures by coming home to an environment of unhappiness or negativity. He needed to be in a nurturing environment, not a hostile one.

In September 1983 Toni passed away the day after leaving our house and being transported to hospital. A very sad time for all concerned, and I think Derek suffered the most of all. He confided in me once that he felt he had failed her and his parents by giving his marrow, which didn't work to fix her. His grief and the grief suffered by my fiancée became destructive to the family unit at times, and a huge barrier to us building healthy relationships all round.

But despite that negative and sad time, we did get married in late October (when my son was two months' old) which had a way of settling everything down to a certain degree. There was some stability and certainty introduced and a "new family" borne of past miseries. Tensions and relationship issues were still highly volatile outside of our immediate family and finances were still tight, but we could at least see positive coming and a chance to build something new together.

After 1984's move of the family to the countryside and long commutes into the city, despite my strong feelings of isolation I did get involved in community activities and returned to full-time work in the city in August 1984. In 1986 I was involved in a fatal motor vehicle accident (MVA) on my way home from being in the city (a Saturday ski-season, fatigue-related crash involving two vehicles ahead of me crashing head on, with multiple injuries to one set of occupants, and fatal injuries for the at-fault driver who'd fallen asleep at the wheel). I was trained in first aid by that stage and attended to the three injured (broken jaw, shock, lacerations type injuries), got them positioned away from their upturned vehicle, turned off ignitions (fuel everywhere on the road meant emergency management procedures had to be actioned), extracted the fatally injured driver sufficiently to clear his airway, however he died of blood loss from his legs and head, and the resultant bodily shock. He died in my arms before the ambulance could arrive.

Somehow I also directed traffic around the scene (we were isolated in the country and not close to emergency services) and, to this day, I have absolutely no idea how I managed to do all of that efficiently in the first 30-40 minutes after the crash. About four hours after the crash and my husband and sons came to pick me up at the scene, I started crying uncontrollably. This was my way of releasing the pressures of that day and not taking the negatives home with me.

Over the years I extended volunteer first aid support to multiple MVAs and was even called by a friend to provide support to some injured people after a bad car wreck on the mountain road above their ranch. My friend's reason was "you always stay so calm". I also attended to the first aid of various motorcycle riders who competed in my son's race meets, over a 7-8 year period. My son was badly hurt one time (multiple fractures and unconscious from a head injury) and many of the riders had serious injuries including one with a broken neck. My approach? Compassionate above all else, but systematic (to manage the risks to those injured). That was a fulfilling time for me; I felt I was doing 'good'.

My grandmother's diagnosis with cancer and her subsequent death in the late 1980's, coupled with the deaths of both my parents-in-law within six weeks of one another, and my mother's diagnosis with cancer, *all within a few months of each other,* simply meant that staying positive was imperative to my and the family's emotional wellbeing. My husband's coping skills were not so good and he suffered a heart attack, cardiac arrest and prolonged ill health and a personality change starting mid 1996. Our separation in early 2001 was actioned by me, but was forseeable as the marriage was going nowhere and the family dynamic was, often times, quite toxic. We divorced in mid 2002.

Whilst I was stalked in the early 2000's by a couple of different men (one of whom I took to court to gain a restraining order), the only other major events that resulted in intense feelings in the moment, were my son reporting yet another serious illness; finding out by accident that my previous partner in the USA was also very ill; and managing a disconnection from the vast majority of my remaining blood relatives on both sides, starting around 2007-8 and completing in 2014 after my mother's death in 2013.

****

All in all, I've had an interesting life full of many lessons! Beyond what I've shared here, there have been other events and situations during my life that have produced all sorts of feelings - sadness, disappointment, annoyance, frustration etc. – but I'm pragmatic in my view that this scenario is the same for most people. The vast majority of us have those times in life when things happen and we don't like or want the new reality that we're facing. In many respects that's just 'life'.

On the other hand, we see some people meander along in life and never really face anything, their lives seeming to track along a smooth, constantly flat path. However, I have often wondered about these folks "what would you have become and how would you have changed if your life had been harder and more challenging?"

This question of mine is founded in the belief I expressed earlier, that people who *are* dished out severe challenges, traumatic events and crises to face are generally more capable of enduring those challenges and thriving afterwards. In my view, life experiences are a gift, and who we become as a result of those experiences; how we choose to treat others despite how we're treated; whether we choose to live lives of integrity and honesty, or malice and revenge, are all a test of our character.

As we choose and as we decide,

so our lives will be formed.

END-NOTE REFERENCES:

i *Dropping the 'D' in PTSD is becoming the norm in Washington*, PowerPost In The Loop, The Washington Post, Colby Itkowitz, June 30, 2015

ii Ibid

iii *Dropping the D is Awesome...What's Next?*, Illinois Fire Fighter Peer Support Blog Post, article by Danielle Fary, on-line posting date July 7, 2015

iv *The day the earth fell on Thredbo*, The Age, on-line post dated July 30, 2002 (www.theage.com.au/articles/2002/07/29/1027926853777.html

v *No Boxing Allowed*, Nola A. Hennessy, ©2009-current, page 50, 92

vi Ibid, page 124

vii www.iso.org

viii American Psychiatric Association at www.psychiatry.org

ix Ibid

x World Health Organization at http://apps.who.int/iris/handle/10665/37108

xi *Mosby's Medical, Nursing and Allied Health Dictionary 4th Edition*, Mosby Year-Book 1994, page 490

xii Ibid, page 490

xiii Ibid, page 542

xiv *ISO 31000:2009 Risk management – Principles and guidelines*

xv *Mosby's Medical, Nursing and Allied Health Dictionary 4th Edition*, Mosby Year-Book 1994, pages 264-276

xvi *Essentials of Anatomy and Physiology*, 4th Edition, Elaine N. Marieb, page 275-276

xvii Ibid, pages 273-276

xviii *Mosby's Medical, Nursing and Allied Health Dictionary 4th Edition*, Mosby Year-Book 1994, page 662

xix Ibid, page 747

xx *Essentials of Anatomy and Physiology*, 4th Edition, Elaine N. Marieb, pages 10-11, 269-276, 307-335, 337, 389, G-10

xxi *Mosby's Fundamentals of Therapeutic Massage*, 1st Edition, Sandy Fritz, page 142

xxii *Essentials of Anatomy and Physiology*, 4th Edition, Elaine N. Marieb, pages 264, G-10

xxiii *Mosby's Medical, Nursing and Allied Health Dictionary 4th Edition*, Mosby Year-Book 1994, page 790

xxiv Ibid, page 790

xxv Ibid, page 823

xxvi Ibid, page 1299

xxvii Ibid, page 1353

xxviii *ISO 31000:2009 Risk management – Principles and guidelines*

xxix *Essentials of Anatomy and Physiology*, 4th Edition, Elaine N. Marieb, page 1491

xxx *Essentials of Anatomy and Physiology*, 4th Edition, Elaine N. Marieb, page G-17

xxxi *Mosby's Medical, Nursing and Allied Health Dictionary 4th Edition*, Mosby Year-Book 1994, page 1515

xxxii Ibid, page 1515

xxxiii Ibid, page 1581

xxxiv Ibid, page 1581

xxxv Ibid, page 1581

xxxvi *Coping with a Major Personal Crisis*, Australian Red Cross (undated c. 1996)

xxxvii *No Boxing Allowed*, Nola A. Hennessy, ©2009-current, page 56

xxxviii Ibid, page 72-73, 75

xxxix *Pain tolerance linked to upbringing: study*, The Canberra Times, May 26, 1998

xl *Gun Violence Takes a Brutal Psychological Toll on Kids*, ABC News, article by Jesse Singal and Avianne Tan, February 17, 2017

xli *Sebastian Junger on post-traumatic stress: 'I just thought I was going crazy'*, The Washington Post, Checkpoint article by Dan Lamothe, May 15, 2015

xlii *Study: For most Vietnam veterans with PTSD, symptoms worse over time*, Stars and Stripes, article by Nancy Montgomery, published on-line July 22, 2015 xliii *NSW: PTSD after collision at sea,* CCH Australia Limited, OHS news article published May 10, 2004

xliv *No Boxing Allowed,* Nola A. Hennessy, ©2009-current, page 110

xlv Ibid, page 67

xlvi Ibid, page 20

xlvii Ibid, page 7

xlviii Ibid, Chapters 4-5, 7-9 and page 36

xlix Ibid, page 36

l *Reason from the heart,* The Canberra Times, article by George Monbiot in London, November 28, 1995

li *Phineas Gage: Neuroscience's Most Famous Patient,* Smithsonian Magazine, article by Steve Swomey, published online January 2010, www.smithsonian.com

lii *Mosby's Medical, Nursing and Allied Health Dictionary 4th Edition,* Mosby Year-Book 1994, page 1353

liii *No Boxing Allowed,* Nola A. Hennessy, ©2009-current, page 75

liv Ibid, page 30

lv Ibid, page 75

lvi Ibid, page 125

lvii Ibid, page 100

lviii Ibid, page 61

www.ingramcontent.com/pod-product-compliance
Lightning Source LLC
Chambersburg PA
CBHW041216030426
42336CB00023B/3359